Medical Lists for Examinations

Medical Lists for Examinations

Second Edition

Roger Gabriel BA, MB, MSc, FRCP, DCH
Renal Physician, St Mary's Hospital, London

Cynthia Gabriel MB, FRCP, DCH
Consultant Paediatrician, St Albans City Hospital and
Queen Elizabeth II Hospital, Welwyn Garden City, Hertfordshire

Butterworths
London Boston Durban Singapore Sydney Toronto Wellington

First published 1983
Reprinted 1985
Second edition 1988

© Butterworth & Co (Publishers) Ltd, 1988

British Library Cataloguing in Publication Data

Gabriel, Roger
  Medical lists for examinations.—2nd ed.
  1. Diseases—Causes and theories of
  causation   2. Symtomatology
  I. Title   II. Gabriel, Cynthia M.
  616.07′1   RB151

  ISBN 0-407-01660-0

Library of Congress Cataloging in Publication Data

Gabriel, Roger.
  Medical lists for examinations/Roger Gabriel,
  Cynthia Gabriel.—2nd ed.
      p.   cm.
  Includes index.
  ISBN 0-407-01660-0   (U.K.)
  1. Internal medicine—Outlines, syllabi, etc.
  2. Medicine—Outlines, syllabi, etc.
  I. Gabriel, Cynthia M.   II. Title.
  [DNLM: 1. Medicine—outlines.   W 18 G118m]
  RC59.G33 1988
  610′.76—dc19
  DNLM/DLC

Photoset by Butterworths Litho Preparation Department
Printed and bound in Great Britain by Anchor Brendon Ltd., Tiptree, Essex

Preface to second edition

The aim of this edition is no different from that of the first. The text has been closely scrutinized and additions and modifications made as necessary. This book contains the information we would have wished to memorize when we read for MB and to act as *aides-mémoire* when studying for College diplomas.

R.G.
C.M.G.

Preface to first edition

This book is a series of lists together with some diagrams and a number of definitions of various medical conditions. It is intended to help those reading for MB and MRCP. No list is exhaustive: we have attempted to avoid obscure conditions and wherever possible the 'causes' are arranged in approximate order of frequency of occurrence. Candidates may be able to find additions to some lists and may search in vain for a section on some favourite topic. The contents of this book will provide a useful framework for revision. We suggest that this book be used by medical students before ward rounds and whilst preparing for finals, and by membership candidates as they read for the College diploma. The text will also be useful for house physicians by suggesting differential diagnoses.

R.G.
C.M.G.

Contents

Abbreviations

AAFB	alcohol-acid fast bacilli	CML	chronic myeloid leukaemia
ACTH	adrenocorticotrophic hormone	CMV	cytomegalovirus
		CNS	central nervous system
ADCC	antibody-dependent cell-mediated cytotoxicity	CREST	calcinosis – Raynaud's phenomenon – (o)esophagus – sclerodactyly telangiectasia (syndrome)
ADH	antidiuretic hormone		
ADP	adenosine diphosphate		
AF	atrial fibrillation	CRF	chronic renal failure
AI	aortic incompetence	CSE	cross-sectional echo
AIDS	acquired immune deficiency syndrome	CSF	cerebrospinal fluid
		CT	computed tomography
AIHA	auto-immune haemolytic anaemia	CVA	cardiovascular accident
		CVS	cardiovascular system
ALA	5-aminolaevulinate	CXR	chest X-ray
ALD	alcoholic liver disease		
ANF	antinuclear factor	DIC	disseminated intravascular coagulation
APTT	activated partial thromboplastin time		
		DU	duodenal ulcer
AR	aortic regurgitation		
ARC	AIDS-related complex	EBV	Epstein–Barr virus
ARDS	adult respiratory distress syndrome	ECG	electrocardiogram
		EEG	electroencephalogram
ARF	acute renal failure	EMG	electromyogram
AS	aortic stenosis	ENA	extractable nuclear antigen
ASD	atrial septal defect	ESR	erythrocyte sedimentation rate
AST	aspartate aminotransferase		
AUC	area under curve		
AV	atrioventricular	FDP	fibrin degeneration products
		FEV	forced expiratory volume
BCG	bacille Calmette-Guérin	FVC	forced vital capacity
CABG	coronary artery bypass grafting	GFR	glomerular filtration rate
		GTT	glucose tolerance test
CAPD	continuous ambulatory peritoneal dialysis	GU	gastric ulcer
		GVH	graft-versus-host (disease)
CGL	chronic granulocytic leukaemia	HAV	hepatitis A virus
		HBV	hepatitis B virus
CHD	coronary heart disease	HDL	high density lipoprotein
CK	creative kinase	HDV	hepatitis D virus
CLL	chronic lymphocytic leukaemia	HIV	human immunodeficiency virus
CMI	cell-mediated immunity		

HLA	human leucocyte antigen	PLG	persistent generalized lymphadenopathy
HSV	herpes simplex virus	PMF	progressive massive fibrosis
ICS	intercostal space	PPD	purified protein derivative (of tuberculin)
ITP	immune thrombocytopenia purpura	PSS	progressive systemic sclerosis
IVC	inferior vena cava	PT	prothrombin time
IVU	intravenous urogram	PTH	parathyroid hormone
		PUO	pyrexia of unknown origin
JCA	juvenile chronic arthritis		
		RA	rheumatoid arthritis
LAD	left anterior descending (artery)	RBB	right bundle branch
		RBBB	right bundle branch block
LAP	left atrial pressure	RBC	red blood corpuscle count
LATS	long-acting thyroid stimulator	RES	reticulo-endothelial system
LBBB	left bundle branch block	RF	rheumatoid factor
LDH	lactate dehydrogenase	RIA	radioimmunoassay
LDL	low density lipoproteins	RICS	right intercostal space
LFT	liver function test	RTA	renal tubular acidosis
LICS	left intercostal space	RVH	right ventricular hypertrophy
LMN	lower motor neurone		
LSE	left sternal edge	SACD	subacute combined degeneration
LVF	left ventricular failure	SAH	subarachnoid haemorrhage
LVH	left ventricular hypertrophy	SBE	subacute bacterial endocarditis
MAP	magnesium – ammonium – phosphate	SCBU	special care baby unit
MCHC	mean corpuscular haemoglobin concentration	SGOT	serum glutamic oxalo-acetic transaminase
MCTD	mixed connective tissue diseases	SIADH	syndrome of inappropriate ADH secretion
MCV	mean corpuscular volume	SLE	systemic lupus erythematosus
MEN	multiple endocrine neoplasia	SVC	superior vena cava
MHC	major histocompatibility complex	TFT	thyroid function test
MI	mitral incompetence	TIBC	total iron-binding capacity
MS	mitral stenosis	TLC	total lung capacity
MSH	melanocyte-stimulating hormone	TNT	trinitrotoluene
		TPN	total parenteral nutrition
NAI	non-accidental injury	TRH	thyrotrophin-releasing hormone
NIDD	non-insulin-dependent (diabetes mellitus)	TSH	thyroid-stimulating hormone
NSAIDs	non-steroidal anti-inflammatory drugs	TT	thrombin time
		UMN	upper motor neurone
PA	postero-anterior	URTI	upper respiratory tract infection
PAN	polyarteritis nodosa	UTI	urinary tract infection
PBG	porphobilinogen		
PCV	packed cell volume	VF	ventricular fibrillation
PDA	patent ductus arteriosus	VLDL	very low density lipoprotein
PE	pulmonary embolism	VSD	ventricular septal defect
PFR	peak flow rate		
PK	pyruvate kinase	WBC	white blood-cell count

Chapter 1

Cardiology

Normal resting intracardiac pressures and saturations

TABLE 1.1

Chamber	Pressure (mmHg)	Oxygen saturation (%)
Right atrium	3–5	
Right ventricle	18/4	
Pulmonary artery	18/12 (mean 15)	65–75
Pulmonary artery wedge	8 (mean)	
Left atrium	8 (mean)	
Left ventricle	130/8	96–98
Aortic root	130/75	

Heart sounds

FIRST SOUND – the abrupt slightly asynchronous closure of the mitral and tricuspid valves.

Loud in:

1. Tachycardia
2. L to R shunts – ASD
3. Mitral stenosis – may be palpable
4. AV dissociation

5/ Short PR Interval

Splits in:

1. Inspiration
2. RBBB

SECOND SOUND – closure of aortic (A2) and pulmonary (P2) valves.

Loud in:

1. Tachycardia
2. Systemic hypertension (A2)

3. Pulmonary hypertension (P2)
4. ASD (P2)

Splits in:

*Wide phys – VSD, M Reg
PV sten, RBBB*

1. Inspiration
2. RBB – widely
3. LBBB – reversed
4. ASD – fixed
5. Pulmonary stenosis

*Rev Split – Aostec LBBB, HOCM
Systemic HT, PDA, LVF
WPW Type B*

THIRD SOUND – shortly after the second sound; caused by rapid filling of the left ventricle. Low frequency.

Heard in:

1. Normal children and adults up to 40 years
2. High atrial pressure from ventricular failure
3. Mitral or tricuspid regurgitation
4. VSD
5. Patent ductus arteriosus

Pericardial Knock in Const Pericard

FOURTH SOUND – immediately before the first sound; caused by atrial contraction. Low frequency.

Heard in:

1. Left ventricular hypertrophy
2. Ischaemic heart disease and hypertension
3. Aortic stenosis

CLICKS – systolic – between first and second sound.

Heard in:

1. Pulmonary hypertension
2. Mitral valve prolapse
3. Bicuspid aortic valve
4. Pulmonary stenosis

OPENING SNAPS – diastolic occurring at the end of opening of mitral and tricuspid valves. High frequency.

Heard in:

1. ASD
2. Mitral stenosis
3. *Tric Stenosis*

Heart sounds

1. Normal
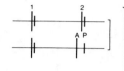
Split first sound; maximum at LSE
Split second sound
P2 less loud than A2

2. Right bundle branch block
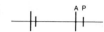
First sound widely split
Second sound widely split – late P2 increases on inspiration

3. Left bundle branch block
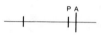
Soft first sound
Second sound reversed splitting due to delay of A2
Maximum in expiration

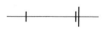
Less on inspiration

4. Third heart sound "Kentucky"
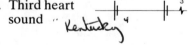
Low frequency

5. Fourth heart sound "Tennessee"
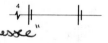
Low frequency

both best heard with patient tipped to left and stethoscope at apex

6. Mitral valve prolapse

Systolic click (sc) best heard at apex when standing

7. Pulmonary hypertension

Early systolic ejection (es) sound at pulmonary area
P2 louder than A2

Heart murmurs

MID-SYSTOLIC EJECTION TYPES

1. Physio-
   logical
   (in youth)

   1-3/6

   Maximal over
   pulmonary area
   Second LICS

2. Aortic
   sclerosis

   2-3/6

   Maximal in aortic,
   LSE and apical
   areas
   Second RICS
   Middle aged and
   elderly

3. Aortic
   stenosis

   es 3-5/6

   Ejection sound
   indicates stenosis;
   disappears with
   rigidity from
   calcium deposition
   First sound is soft
   Second sound
   single or may be
   reversed and A2
   soft with valve
   calcification

4. Obstructive
   cardio-
   myopathy

   2-5/6

   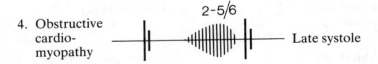

   Late systole

5. Pulmonary
   stenosis

   es   3-5/6   A P

   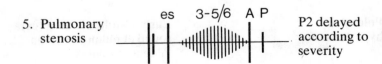

   P2 delayed
   according to
   severity

PANSYSTOLIC REGURGITANT TYPES

1. Mitral regurgitation

2-5/6   A P

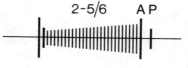

Long murmur tends to drown A2 May be wide split of second sounds A short diastolic murmur may occur from rapid ventricular filling If with mitral stenosis, the murmer is longer and less abrupt

2. Tricuspid regurgitation

2-4/6

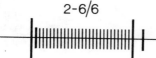

Best heard at LSE, fourth ICS and usually accompanied by systolic liver expansion and a jugular venous wave

3. Ventricular septal defect – VSD

2-6/6

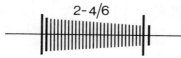

The murmur may be absent with larger defects A flow ejection systolic murmur may also be present over the aortic area Best heard at LSE

GRADES OF MURMURS

1. Just audible
2. Quiet
3. Moderate
4. Loud with thrill
5. Very loud with thrill
6. Audible without stethoscope

DIASTOLIC MURMURS

1. Mitral stenosis

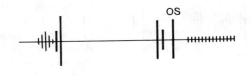

The length of the diastolic murmur is proportional to the severity of the stenosis
Mid-diastolic and apical presystolic murmur if in sinus rhythm

2. Atrial septal defect – ASD

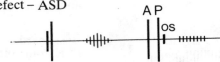

The diastolic murmur is caused by blood flowing from the L atrium across the ASD to the R atrium

3. Aortic or pulmonary regurgitation

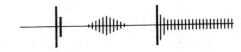

High frequency decrescendo murmur
The systolic murmur is caused by the increased ventricular stroke volume

Mitral regurgitation (incompetence; MI)

Competence depends on the left atrial wall, mitral annulus, valve leaflets, chordae tendineae, papillary muscles and left ventricle.

CAUSES

1. Floppy prolapsing valve
2. Rheumatic – usually with some stenosis
3. Papillary muscle dysfunction – ischaemia or inferior infarction
4. Bacterial endocarditis – either on a previously abnormal valve or spread from an infected aortic valve
5. Secondary to left ventricular dilatation in heart failure
6. Cardiomyopathy (HOCM) – papillary muscle malalignment
7. Congenital – rare; most commonly with a primum ASD

COMPLICATIONS

1. Often none
2. Atrial fibrillation ⎫ less frequently than in
3. Systemic emboli ⎬ patients with mitral
4. Bronchitis ⎭ stenosis
5. LVF
6. SBE

Mitral stenosis (MS)

CAUSES

1. Rheumatic
2. Congenital – very rare *Lutembacher's sy*   MS + ASD

COMPLICATIONS

1. Atrial fibrillation – due to atrial dilatation; occurs in virtually all patients
2. Systemic emboli – in 20 per cent
3. Functional tricuspid incompetence and right heart failure following uncontrolled AF
4. Pulmonary hypertension – in about 25 per cent of patients
5. Bronchitis
6. Haemoptysis
7. SBE – uncommon

Tricuspid incompetence

ACQUIRED

1. Functional – secondary to RV dilatation caused by pulmonary hypertension
2. Following SBE – usually in 'main-lining' drug addicts
3. Carcinoid syndrome – in 50 per cent of cases; rare
4. Rheumatic – rarely isolated; infrequent

CONGENITAL – Ebstein's anomaly

Aortic stenosis (AS)

1. Calcification of a congenitally bicuspid valve
2. Rheumatic (often with AI)
3. Degenerative – calcification, progressing from aortic sclerosis

Assoc. Coarct of Ao

4. Congenital – may present first in adult life
5. Supravalvular stenosis ⎱ infrequent; haemodynamically
6. Subvalvular obstruction ⎰ the same as for aortic stenosis

COMPLICATIONS

1. Angina – may occur with normal coronary arteries
2. Dyspnoea – LVF
3. Syncope – of exertion or ventricular arrhythmia
4. Sudden death in 10–20 per cent

Aortic incompetence or regurgitation (AI, AR)

CHRONIC

1. Rheumatic – about 50 per cent of patients; often with AS
2. SBE – usually on a previously abnormal valve
3. Severe hypertension
4. Syphilitic
5. Congenital
6. Seronegative arthritides:
   i. ankylosing spondylitis ⎱ rare
   ii. Reiter's syndrome
7. Cystic medial necrosis – Marfan's   ← *NBM – Cardiac problem in homocystinuria*

ACUTE – presents as sudden pulmonary oedema

1. SBE – perforation of a valve cusp
2. Dissecting aneurysm of ascending aorta
3. Deceleration trauma

Bradycardia

Ventricular rate <60 beats per minute (arbitrary) due to dysfunction of the heart muscle or conduction tissues.

1. Sinus bradycardia
   i.   normal people asleep
   ii. athletes – high vagal tone
   iii. beta-adrenergic blocking drugs
   iv. in first 24–48 hours of myocardial infarction
   v.   digoxin
   vi. myxoedema
   vii. jaundice

2. Sinus arrest – cessation of sinus node for 2 seconds or more
3. Sinoatrial block – impaired conduction of depolarizing wave from sinoatrial node
4. The above abnormalities may be complicated by:
   i.   junctional rhythms
   ii. frequent extrasystoles – atrial or ventricular ectopic beats
   iii. supraventricular or ventricular tachycardias
5. 2:1 or 3:1 AV block
6. Complete heart block

Heart block

TYPES

1. First degree – prolonged PR interval (>0.2 seconds), no symptoms or signs
2. Second degree – dropped beats – some P waves fail to conduct to ventricles
   i. Mobitz Type I – progressive lengthening of the PR inter-
       (Wenckebach)   vals until an impulse is not transmitted. After a pause the QRS starts again immediately following a normal P wave
   ii. Mobitz Type II – PR interval of conducted beats is constant. Periodic failure of conduction of impulse from atrium to ventricle. Lesion below the bifurcation of the bundle of His
3. Third degree – complete block. No relationship between atrial and ventricular complexes
4. Bundle branch block – diagnostic features:
   i.   widening of the QRS to 0.12 seconds or more
   ii. distortion of the QRS to produce an RSR′, rSR′ or rsR′ pattern due to a 'late' R wave over the branch blocked ventricle
   iii. ST segment depression and T-wave inversion over the blocked ventricle
   Right, left, left anterior and left posterior hemiblocks are recognized

Causes of complete heart block

ACUTE

1. Myocardial infarction – usually an anterior infarct
2. Infections causing carditis – rheumatic, diphtheria, viral and bacterial endocarditis

CHRONIC

1. Degeneration (presumably ischaemic) of the conducting fibres
2. Subsequent to myocardial infarct – infrequent as the acute block either resolves or is fatal

Causes of right bundle branch block

1. Congenital – asymptomatic, normal life expectation
2. Ischaemic heart disease – most common
3. Pulmonary hypertension
4. Pulmonary embolism
5. Rate dependent – present only during a tachycardia
6. Associated with an ASD – ostium secundum
7. Following cardiac surgery

Causes of left bundle branch block

Always pathological with a serious prognosis.

1. Ischaemic heart disease – the most common
2. Left ventricular hypertrophy – all causes
3. Aortic stenosis with calcium deposition extending to the conducting system
4. Cardiomyopathy
5. Following cardiac surgery

Tachycardias

SINUS TACHYCARDIAS

Rate 100–200 beats/minute

1. Anxiety
2. Fever
3. Congestive heart failure
4. Hypovolaemia – severe bleeding
5. Vasodilator drugs – hydralazine, nitrites, minoxidil
6. Constrictive pericarditis – rare

ATRIAL ARRHYTHMIAS

1. Atrial ectopics
2. Atrial fibrillation – atrial rate 350–600, ventricular rate 60–200
    i.   thyrotoxicosis
    ii. ischaemic heart disease

   iii. rheumatic heart disease
   iv. idiopathic – 'lone'
   v. pericarditis – constrictive or infiltrating neoplasm
   vi. cardiomyopathy
3. Atrial flutter – rate 260–320, ventricular rate 80–300, regular
4. Supraventricular tachycardia – rapidly discharging atrial focus; atrial rate 160–210, ventricular rate 160–210, regular

VENTRICULAR TACHYCARDIAS

1. Ventricular tachycardia – rate 120–250; most frequently postinfarction
2. Paroxysmal ventricular tachycardia
   i. thyrotoxicosis
   ii. digitalis poisoning
   iii. hypokalaemia
3. Ventricular fibrillation – rate >250; very common postinfarction. Spontaneous self-limiting runs of VF occur in hypothermia

Complications of acute myocardial infarction

EARLY

1. Sudden death – 30–50 per cent of patients
2. Haemodynamic changes:
   i. hypotension
   ii. pulmonary congestion – 50 per cent
   iii. pulmonary oedema – 5–10 per cent
   iv. oliguria
   v. hypoxaemia – impaired diffusion and shunting
   vi. hypocapnia – mild, caused by hyperventilation
   vii. cardiogenic shock – any three of the following:
      (a) hypotension – systolic pressure <90 mmHg
      (b) oliguria
      (c) cold, clammy skin
      (d) mental confusion
      (e) metabolic acidosis
3. Arrhythmias – any type may occur. Most common are:
   i. ventricular ectopics – the most common
   ii. atrial flutter or fibrillation – 15–25 per cent
   iii. ventricular tachycardia
   iv. heart block

    v. ventricular fibrillation – most common in the first hour postinfarction

4. Mitral incompetence occurs in up to 20 per cent and is mild and transient – papillary muscle dysfunction
5. Pericarditis – in about 25 per cent with transmural infarction
6. Cardiac rupture

    i. into pericardium – no pulse, ECG maintained for 15–30 minutes

    ii. through septum – L to R shunt, VSD

LATER

1. Deep venous thrombosis and pulmonary embolism
2. Mural thrombi and systemic emboli
3. Dressler's syndrome – postmyocardial infarction syndrome
4. Frozen shoulder
5. Left ventricular aneurysm

Prognosis after acute myocardial infarction

PROGNOSTICALLY POOR FEATURES

1. Past history of a previous infarct
2. Signs of left ventricular failure
3. Cardiomegaly
4. Anteroseptal infarction

    i. conduction system is located primarily at this site

    ii. anterior infarcts have up to twice the mortality of inferior infarcts

5. RBBB with an anterior infarct or a bifascicular block – RBBB with left anterior hemiblock
6. Ventricular arrhythmias late in the admission
7. Late postinfarct angina
8. Left ventricular thrombi
9. ST segment depression on exercise testing – a strong predictor of future cardiac events
10. Poor rise in systolic pressure on testing ⎱ indicate latent
11. Inappropriate tachycardia at low exercise load ⎰ myocardial dysfunction
12. Persistent cigarette smoking
13. Persistent heavy drinking of alcohol

Diagnostic criteria for myocardial infarction

DEFINITE INFARCTION

1. Typical ischaemic pain history
2. Q waves or sequential ST segment and T wave changes, or both
3. Rise in concentration of cardiac enzymes to more than twice the upper limit of normal

POSSIBLE INFARCTION

1. Typical pain
2. ECG not typical
3. Cardiac enzymes not raised above twice the upper limit of normal

Causes of chest pain

1. Ischaemic heart disease – infarction and angina
2. Oesophagitis } both posture related
3. Pericarditis }
4. Pleurisy
5. Structural lesions of nerve roots or ribs
6. Oesophageal spasm

Pain with breathlessness

1. Angina with transient lung congestion
2. Pleuritic or pericardial pain limiting respiratory excursion
3. Pleuritic pain with pneumonia or pulmonary embolism

Sudden onset of dyspnoea at rest

1. Left heart failure
2. Pneumothorax
3. Pulmonary embolism
4. Asthma
5. Acute pneumonia
6. Sudden occlusion of a large airway

Indications for pacing

TEMPORARY PACING

1. Acute third degree block complicating myocardial infarction
2. Long PR interval with new RBBB and left anterior or posterior hemiblock

3. Alternating RBBB and LBBB
4. Tachyarrhythmias resistant to drug treatment
5. Postcardiac surgery
6. Overdose of digoxin or β-blockers

PERMANENT PACING

1. Chronic AV block with Stokes–Adams attacks
2. Patients with symptomatic bradyarrhythmias
3. Sick sinus syndrome – variable abnormal periods of atrial discharges; demand pacing employed in selected patients

Causes of an irregular pulse

1. Sinus arrhythmia – young, elderly, postinfarct
2. Ventricular or supraventricular extrasystoles – common
3. Atrial fibrillation
4. Atrial flutter with varying block

Heart muscle disease

ACUTE MYOCARDITIS

All uncommon in Western Europe.

1. Infections – viral (echovirus), or bacterial (diphtheria)
2. Acute rheumatic fever
3. Lead poisoning
4. X-irradiation
5. Drugs
   i.   doxorubicin } cumulative poisons
   ii. daunorubicin
   iii. alcohol induced

CARDIOMYOPATHIES

Classification according to effects on ventricular function. Causes unknown. Defined as heart muscle diseases of unknown cause.

1. Congestive (dilated) – poor systolic contraction and high end-diastolic volume
2. Hypertrophic (HOCM) – ventricular muscle hypertrophy impairing diastolic filling with or without outflow tract obstruction
3. Restrictive – a stiffened myocardium leading to impaired filling of ventricles. Similar to constrictive pericarditis

SPECIFIC HEART MUSCLE DISEASE

1. Amyloid ⎫
2. Sarcoid ⎬ congestive
3. Haemochromatosis ⎱ cardiomyopathies
4. Secondary haemosiderosis ⎭
5. Progressive systemic sclerosis

Pericarditis

The majority of these conditions may present without an effusion and later develop an effusion.

1. Acute idiopathic
2. Acute transmural myocardial infarction
3. Postmyocardial, postcardiotomy and traumatic
4. Uraemia – usually preterminal
5. Malignant infiltration of pericardium
6. Collagen diseases – SLE especially
7. Infections – tuberculosis*, bacterial, viral, fungal, parasitic
8. Radiotherapy*
9. Drug-induced – hydralazine, procainamide
10. Myxoedema

Haemopericardium

1. Trauma – penetrating and non-penetrating
2. Advanced uraemia
3. Dissecting aortic aneurysm
4. Bleeding diathesis – leukaemias
5. Rupture of ventricle
6. Myxoedema

Signs of tamponade

Raised pressure in the pericardium impairing ventricular filling

1. Tachycardia
2. Paradoxical pulse
3. Elevated venous pressure without the inspiratory rise
4. Decreased blood pressure
5. Faintness, dyspnoea
6. No murmurs

* may lead to constrictive pericarditis

Left ventricular failure (LVF)

CLINICAL TRIAD

1. Triple rhythm – atrial or third heart sound
2. Pulsus alternans – alternate large and small beats
3. Basal crepitations – pulmonary oedema

CAUSES

1. Disease of left ventricle
   i.   ischaemia – the most common cause
   ii. hypertrophic obstructive cardiomyopathy – infrequent
   iii. myocarditis
2. Pressure (systolic) load
   i.   hypertension – common
   ii. aortic stenosis
3. Volume (diastolic) load
   i.   aortic incompetence
   ii. mitral incompetence
   iii. left to right shunts – VSD, patent ductus

Right ventricular failure

1. Secondary to (systolic pressure load)
   i.   cor pulmonale – the most common – or thromboembolism
   ii. persistent LVF – common
   iii. mitral stenosis
   iv. pulmonary fibrosis
   v.   ASD
2. Isolated disease of the right heart – pulmonary stenosis–rare

Causes of pulmonary hypertension

1. Chronic bronchitis – hypoxic vasoconstriction
2. Left heart disease
   i.   left ventricular failure
   ii. mitral stenosis
3. Pulmonary embolism – *see* page 29
4. Left to right shunts – ASD, VSD, PDA
5. Pulmonary fibrosis – occupational lung disease – *see* page 49
6. Idiopathic

Cor pulmonale

Hypertrophy and dilatation of right ventricle as a result of lung disease   Long term ↓ PO_2

1. Diseases of airways and lung parenchyma
   i. chronic bronchitis ⎫ easily the most common
   ii. emphysema   ⎬
   iii. pulmonary infiltrations and granulomata
   iv. cystic fibrosis
   v. lung fibrosis
2. Disorders of thoracic cage
   i. severe kyphoscoliosis – when deformity angle greater than 100 degrees
   ii. large thoracoplasty – now uncommon
3. Pulmonary vascular disease
   i. pulmonary emboli
   ii. schistosomiasis – common in tropical areas
   iii. primary – very rare
4. Neuromuscular disease
   i. poliomyelitis
   ii. myasthenia gravis
   iii. amyotrophic lateral sclerosis
   iv. muscular dystrophy and myopathies
5. Respiratory control disturbance
   i. idiopathic hypoventilation
   ii. obesity (>130 kg) – hypoventilation syndrome
   iii. cerebrovascular disease
6. Obstruction of extrathoracic airways–tonsils and adenoids in children

Unfavourable factors for valve surgery

1. Myocardial dysfunction
2. Concurrent coronary artery disease
3. Abnormal lung function
4. Concurrent peripheral arterial disease
5. Renal or hepatic impairment

Long-term complications of valve replacement

1. Valve failure   ⎫ these risks differ greatly
2. Myocardial failure   ⎪ with the prosthesis,
3. Thromboembolism   ⎬ the implantation site and
4. Prosthetic endocarditis ⎭ the original disease

Long-term results of aortic valve replacement with a mechanical valve are usually first class; success is less assured with mitral and multiple valve replacements.

Infective endocarditis

Usually a mild valvular incompetence is the site of the infection; less often a septal defect or the mural endocardium of a ventricular aneurysm. Endocarditis is most likely to occur when blood jets from a high to a low pressure chamber. Has a 30 per cent mortality rate which is not improving.

1. Medical
    i.   *Streptococcus viridans* strains – 80 per cent
    ii. *Enterococcus* strains – 10 per cent

2. Elderly
    i.   *Strep. viridans* – 50 per cent
    ii. *Strep. faecalis*
    iii. Gram negative bacteria

3. Cardiac surgery
    i.   *Staph. epidermidis* and *aureus*
    ii. *Candida albicans*

4. Narcotic addicts – often the tricuspid valve is affected
    i.   *Staph. aureus*
    ii. *Serratia marcescens*
    iii. multiple infections in some

5. Culture negative
    i.   up to 20 per cent of cases
    ii. often previous antibiotic drugs
    iii. Coxiella or Chlamydia

1. Dental procedures
2. Urinary catheterization
3. D and C — all allowing low virulence bacteria
4. Cardiac surgery — access to the circulation
5. Bed sores
6. Haemodialysis
7. Increasing number of invasive diagnostic and therapeutic procedures

Cardiac 'queer' turns

1. Fainting
2. Carotid sinus syncope – tight collars in the elderly
3. Cardiac arrhythmias
   i.   heart block – Stokes–Adams attack ⎱ with fall
   ii. sick sinus syndrome   ⎰ in cardiac
   iii. paroxysmal tachycardia   output
4. Ventricular outflow obstruction
   i.   HOCM   ⎱ exertional syncope
   ii. aortic stenosis ⎰
5. Drugs
   i.   causing conduction disturbances
        (a) antiarrhythmics
        (b) β-blockers
        (c) digoxin
   ii. vasodilators
        (a) first dose effect of prazosin and angiotensin converting
            enzyme inhibitors
        (b) hydralazine
        (c) glyceryl trinitrate
   iii. causing arrhythmias
        (a) tricyclic antidepressants
        (b) digoxin
6. Pacemakers
   i.   technical failures
   ii. external interference

Indications for endomyocardial biopsy

1. Diagnosis and management of rejection after cardiac transplant
2. Myocarditis   ⎱ of unknown origin
3. Congestive heart failure ⎰

Chapter 2
Electrocardiography

The normal ECG trace

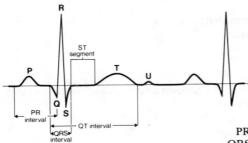

Figure 2.1

PR interval   0.12–0.20 seconds
QRS interval   0.07–0.10 seconds
ST segment   0.14–0.16 seconds
QT interval   0.33–0.43 seconds
PR, QT, and RR intervals vary with the heart rate

$$QT_c = \frac{QT}{\sqrt{RR}}$$

Ventricular hypertrophy – ECG criteria

LVH

1. Large R in I, aVL, V5 and V6 >30 mm in V5 or V6
2. Large S in V1 or V2 >30 mm
3. Inverted T and depressed ST in leads with a large R wave

ELECTRICAL CRITERIA FOR LVH

S in V1 or V2 + R in V5 or V6 = >35 mm

RVH

1. Dominant R in V1 or V2 – essential
2. Prominent S in I, aVL, V5 or V6
3. Inverted T and depressed ST in leads with dominant R

20

ECG signs of transmural infarction

TABLE 2.1

ST elevation – convex upwards in leads, over infarcted area	Lasts 3–4 days If persistent indicates aneurysm of ventricle Reciprocal ST depression in leads over areas opposite to infarct
T wave inversion – over the infarct	May disappear in a few months, but may remain indefinitely
Q wave >2 mm deep over infarct	Permanent

Changes in the ST segment

TABLE 2.2

Elevation	Other features
1. Transmural infarction – convex upward	See above
2. Early pericarditis – convex downward	T wave inversion later
3. Hypothermia	Clinical features, J waves, slow heart, increased PR, QRS and QT intervals
4. LV aneurysm	Characteristic QRS changes
5. LVH or RVH	
6. Early repolarization pattern – convex upward	Tall and peaked T waves
7. RBBB or LBBB	Characteristic QRS complexes

TABLE 2.3

Depression	Other features
1. Transient ischaemia	Revert to normal quickly. Angina
2. Subendocardial infarction	Often with inverted T waves over infarct
3. Hypokalaemia	U waves may be present. T waves flattened
4. Digitalis – concave upwards	Flattened or inverted T. QT interval shortened
5. LVH or RVH	} Characteristic QRS configuration
6. RBBB or LBBB	

Causes of T wave inversion or flattening

1. Transient ischaemia
2. Transmural infarction
3. Subendothelial infarction
4. Pericarditis – later stages
5. Hypokalaemia
6. Digitalis
7. LVH or RVH
8. RBBB or LBBB
9. Persistent juvenile pattern

Potassium and ECG changes

TABLE 2.4

	K ↑ >7.5 mmol/ℓ	K ↓ <2 mmol/ℓ
P	Flat	Prolonged
R	Flattened	
QRS	Widened	
ST segment		Depressed
T	Tall, peaked and broader – especially mid-precordial leads	Flat or inverted
U		Prominent – especially in mid-precordial leads
Later changes	Sine wave, ventricular tachycardia and fibrillation	

Potassium, calcium and ECG changes

TABLE 2.5

	K ↑	K ↓	Ca²⁺ ↑	Ca²⁺ ↓
Early changes	Tall, peaked T	Large U	QT interval ↓	QT interval ↑
Late features	Flattened P and R Broadened QRS Sine wave Arrhythmias	Flattened or inverted T ST depressed	More pronounced	More pronounced

Ectopic beats

1. Atrial – P' followed by a normal QRS. The P' may resemble a sinus P
2. Junctional – retrograde P' proceeding, following or hidden within a normal QRS
3. Ventricular – wide and bizarre QRS. The QRS complex is similar to:

   i. QRS or RBBB if impulse originates in LV or,
   ii. LBBB if impulse originates in RV

Ventricular ectopic rhythms

TABLE 2.6

	Rate	ECG
Ventricular tachycardia	100–250/minute regular	Abrupt onset and cessation. Sinus P waves independent of ventricular activity. QRS configuration like that of an isolated ventricular ectopic beat
Ventricular fibrillation	Rapid and irregular	Irregular and continuously varying trace. Terminal
Ventricular escape rhythm: idioventricular	35–40/minute regular	As for ventricular tachycardia. Third degree block
Accelerated idioventricular rhythm	50–100/minute regular	As for ventricular tachycardia

Myocardial infarction

TABLE 2.7

	Anteroseptal (anterior)	Anterolateral (lateral)	Inferior	True posterior
ECG changes	Sequentially – ST ↑, inverted T, abnormal Q in I, aVL, V1–3	Sequentially – ST ↑, inverted T, abnormal Q in I, aVL, V5–6	Sequentially – ST ↑, inverted T, abnormal Q in II, III, aVF	Large, often dominant R in V1 and V2
Reciprocal changes	Depressed ST in II, III, aVF	Depressed ST in II, III, aVF	Depressed ST in I, aVL, V1–3	Nil

Dominant R in V1–2

1. Right ventricular hypertrophy
   i. pulmonary hypertension ⎫
   ii. pulmonary embolism ⎭ strain
2. RBBB
3. True posterior infarct
4. HOCM
5. Type A Wolff–Parkinson–White syndrome

Extracardiac factors affecting the ECG

PHARMACOLOGICAL

1. Negative inotropics
2. Atropine
3. Catecholamines
4. Tricyclic antidepressants

PATHOLOGICAL

1. Myxoedema
2. Cerebrovascular accidents
3. Hypothermia
4. $K^+ \uparrow$ or $K^+ \downarrow$
5. $Ca^{2+} \uparrow$ or $Ca^{2+} \downarrow$
6. Infectious fevers
7. Chest deformities
8. Muscular dystrophy – rare

Echocardiography

Ultrasound waves pass poorly through the lung: hence the beam is limited to a small area of chest wall around the left sternal edge where the heart is not covered by lung. In M-mode echocardiography a single ultrasound beam is directed towards the heart from the fourth or fifth LICS. High definition records are obtained allowing accurate measurements, but the beam is narrow (1–2 cm) allowing only a small part of the heart to be examined at a time. Two-dimensional (2-D; cross-sectional echo, CSE) echocardiography uses multiple beams resulting in a moving picture. The 2-D technique delineates complex anatomical relationships, but at the cost of precise timing and accuracy. M-mode is much cheaper and more widely available than 2-D echocardiography.

Either technique reliable in:
1. Aortic or mitral regurgitation
2. Left atrial enlargement

M-mode superior in:
1. Left ventricular hypertrophy
2. Left ventricular filling rate (assessment of mitral stenosis)
3. Mitral valve vibrations or closure (as in aortic regurgitation)
4. Pericardial effusion

2-D superior in:
1. Direct measurement of mitral and aortic valve areas
2. Aortic root dissection
3. Regional variations of left ventricular function

Exercise electrocardiography

APPLICATIONS

1. Evaluation of ischaemic heart disease
2. Assessment of prognosis in:
   i.   asymptomatic patients
   ii. subjects with coronary artery disease
   iii. following myocardial infarction
3. Assessment postmyocardial revascularization
4. Provocation of arrhythmias

CONTRAINDICATIONS

1. Unstable angina
2. Myocardial infarction <7 days old   } absolute
3. Severe aortic stenosis
4. Severe pulmonary hypertension
5. Physical infirmity   } relative
6. Lack of co-ordination or ataxia

INDICATIONS FOR STOPPING EXERCISE TESTING

1. Ventricular tachycardia
2. Falling blood pressure   } absolute
3. Deteriorating physical condition
4. ST depression >4 mm   } relative
5. Other rhythm disturbances

Chapter 3

Cardiovascular medicine

Blood volume, pressure and flow

Volume in normal adults	5 ℓ (haematocrit 45 per cent)
Central volume (heart and lungs)	1.5 ℓ
Heart blood volume	0.6 ℓ
Left ventricular end-diastolic volume	140 ml
Stroke volume	90 ml
End-systolic volume	50 ml
Ejection fraction	50–70 per cent

$$\text{Mean arterial pressure} = \text{diastolic pressure} + \frac{\text{pulse pressure}}{3}$$

Arterial hypertension

1. Essential – primary; 85–90 per cent of patients
2. Renal

   i. parenchymal ischaemia $\Big\}$ fairly common
   ii. chronic renal failure

3. Vascular

   i. coarctation – upper half of body $\Big\}$ rare
   ii. renal artery stenosis

4. Hormonal

   i. oral contraceptives – fairly common
   ii. Cushing's disease
   iii. primary aldosteronism – Conn's $\Big\}$ rare. Cumulatively all together comprise <1 per cent of hypertensive patients
   iv. phaeochromocytoma
   v. acromegaly

5. Toxaemia of pregnancy – fairly common

Causes of raised plasma noradrenaline

Normal <1 ng/ml

1. 'Shock'
   i. septicaemic
   ii. hypovolaemic
   iii. cardiogenic
2. Postmyocardial infarct
3. Congestive cardiac failure
4. Diabetic ketoacidosis
5. Subarachnoid haemorrhage
6. Phaeochromocytoma – very rare

Risk factors for coronary heart disease (CHD)

PRIMARY INDEPENDENT FACTORS

1. Hypercholesterolaemia ⎤ each factor is of
2. Hypertension   ⎬ approximately equal
3. Cigarette smoking   ⎦ importance

SECONDARY RISK FACTORS

1. Reduced HDL cholesterol concentration ⎤ less
2. Obesity   consistently
3. Insulin dependent diabetes   demonstrated
4. Family history of CHD   ⎬ or may be
5. Physical inactivity   mediated by
6. Stress and personality type   the primary
7. Gout and hyperuricaemia   ⎦ factors
8. Increasing age

UNCERTAIN RISK FACTORS

1. Water hardness
2. Fibre intake

Risk factors for cerebral infarction

ESTABLISHED

1. Age
2. Hypertension
3. Heart disease
4. Atrial fibrillation

5. Diabetes mellitus
6. Transient ischaemic attacks
7. Peripheral vascular disease
8. Oral contraceptive pill

POSSIBLE

1. Cigarette smoking
2. Hyperlipidaemia
3. Obesity
4. Lack of exercise

Arterial disease of the legs

CHRONIC

1. Atherosclerosis – medium and large arteries
2. Buerger's disease – thromboangiitis obliterans
3. Popliteal artery occlusion
4. Small artery occlusion

ACUTE

1. Arterial embolism
2. Acute thrombosis – on an atheromatous plaque
3. Arterial trauma
4. Dissecting aneurysm
5. Frostbite

Pathogenesis of venous thrombi

1. Decreased rate of blood flow
   i.   bed rest
   ii. obstruction to flow – prolonged sitting or pillows under calves
   iii. slow circulation as in heart failure
2. Damage to intima of vein
   i.   trauma and operations
   ii. childbirth
3. Enhanced coagulability
   i.   oral contraceptives
   ii. malignant disease
   iii. dehydration
   iv. polycythaemia
   v.   diabetes mellitus

Pulmonary embolism (PE)

TABLE 3.1

Features	Acute massive PE	Acute minor PE	Chronic thrombo-embolic pulmonary hypertension
Symptoms	Acute dyspnoea, collapse	Pleurisy Haemoptysis	Pleurisy } Recurrent Haemoptysis } Progressive dyspnoea
Signs	Low cardiac output Right ventricular failure	Pain Tachypnoea	Severe pulmonary hypertension
ECG	$S_1Q_3T_3$ pattern RV strain RBBB	Normal	Right axis deviation RVH
CXR	Asymmetrical oligaemia	Pulmonary infarct or normal	Dilatation of pulmonary artery Asymmetrical oligaemia
Pulmonary arteriography	Complete obstruction of parts of the pulmonary tree Reduced filling of peripheral vessels	Not indicated	Dilated central arteries with asymmetrical perfusion of the lung fields

Dissecting aortic aneurysm

SITES

1. Ascending aorta extending to thoracic and abdominal aorta – most common
2. Confined to the ascending aorta – second most frequent
3. Beginning in the descending portion and extending to the abdominal aorta

CAUSES

1. Isolated cystic medial necrosis of aortic wall – the most common
2. Complicating an atherosclerotic aneurysm
3. As part of Marfan's syndrome
4. Complicating coarctation or systemic hypertension

Aortic aneurysm

ASCENDING AORTA

Causes

1. Atheroma – 75 per cent
2. Cystic medial necrosis – 20 per cent
3. Syphilis <5 per cent

} sinuses of Valsalva involved in 10 per cent; asymptomatic in 10 per cent; chest X-ray (*see* page 59)

DESCENDING AORTA

Causes

1. Atheroma – the major cause; usually asymptomatic
2. Trauma

Misdiagnosis of angina

Because of
1. Unusual site of pain
2. Discomfort or breathlessness > pain
3. May be dependent on cold or a meal
4. May be excitement induced
5. The known presence of another cause of the symptom – gall stones, cervical spondylitis, hiatus hernia

Misdiagnosis of a myocardial infarction

1. Painless
2. Associated with an arrhythmia, CVA or syncope
3. Unusual site of pain
4. Normal ECG
5. Patient not ill

Possible indications for β-blockade

1. Hypertension
2. Angina pectoris
3. Following myocardial infarction
4. Arrhythmias
5. HOCM
6. Thyrotoxicosis
7. Anxiety and tremor
8. Migraine
9. Phaeochromocytoma – α-blockade also required

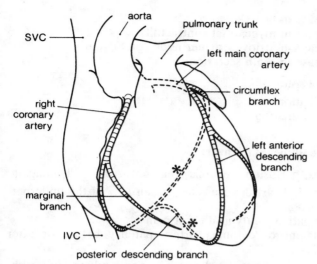

Figure 3.1 The coronary arteries. Anastomotic areas are shown by asterisks. The left anterior descending (LAD) artery is the single most important vessel because it supplies the anterior aspects of both ventricles and is often affected by atheroma.

Indications for coronary arteriography

1. Anginal pain refractory to full medical therapy
2. When there is a need to establish or exclude patency
3. Unstable angina ⎫
4. Evolving myocardial infarction ⎬ underevaluation

Indications for coronary artery bypass grafting (CABG)

1. Relief of refractory angina
2. Obstruction (80 per cent or more) to:
   i. LAD branch
   ii. left main branch
   iii. proximal obstruction to at least two major arteries

   Disease affecting the R main artery or circumflex artery alone is not an indication for surgery.

3. Selected patients with unstable angina

Effects of adrenoceptor stimulation

1. α-adrenoceptors – vasoconstriction
2. β_1-adrenoceptors –

   i.   increase in heart rate
   ii. increase in myocardial contractility
   iii. increase in atrioventricular node conduction
   iv. increase in renin secretion

3. β_2-adrenoceptors –
   i.   vasodilation
   ii. bronchodilation

Radionuclide studies of the heart

1. Myocardial perfusion – exercise thallium–201 (^{201}Tl) imaging
   i.   ischaemic heart disease – to gain an idea of the underper-
        fused areas
   ii. investigation of atypical chest pain
   iii. assessment of coronary artery patency before or after
        CABG
2. Ventricular function – radionuclide ventriculography; tech-
   netium–99m (^{99m}Tc) labelling of the patient's red blood cells
   i.   assessment and detection of ischaemic heart disease using
        measurement of decrease in ejection fraction with stress –
        dynamic, cold pressor or isometric
   ii. assessment of ventricular response to drugs
   iii. diagnosis of ventricular aneurysms
   iv. assessment of ventricular function before and after CABG
3. Measuring shunts   ⎫
4. Chamber filling sequence – used in some   ⎬ ^{99m}Tc used
   paediatric patients   ⎭

Postural (orthostatic) hypotension

DEFINITION

Inability to compensate by increasing peripheral vascular resistance for venous pooling and fall in cardiac output which result
from standing. A fall in systolic pressure by 30 mmHg or to below
80 mmHg.

SHORT LIVED

1. Sodium depletion
2. Drugs – guanethidine, labetalol

CHRONIC ASYMPATHETIC DYSFUNCTION

Supersensitivity to α- or β-sympathomimetics is present

1. Diabetes mellitus – easily the most common
2. Idiopathic Parkinsonism
3. Lesions at the following sites
   i. pyramidal
   ii. extrapyramidal
   iii. cerebellar
4. Rheumatoid arthritis
5. Chronic tetraplegics
6. Multiple system atrophy – Shy–Drager syndrome
7. Hyperbradykinaemia – very rare
8. Idiopathic

TREATMENT OF CHRONIC FORMS

1. Antigravity garments
2. Tilting of bed foot-up
3. 9α-fluoro-hydrocortisone
4. Sympathomimetic amines and perhaps β-blockers

Chapter 4

Chest diseases

Spirometry

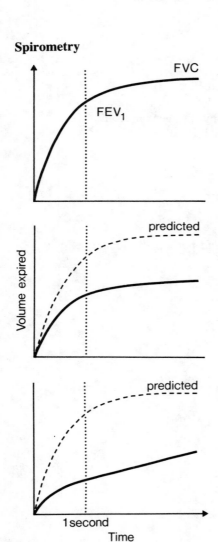

NORMAL

$$\frac{FEV_1}{FVC} = >70 \text{ per cent}$$

RESTRICTIVE DEFECT (FEV_1 AND VC REDUCED COMPARABLY)

$$\frac{FEV_1}{FVC} = >70 \text{ per cent}$$

Causes
1. Fibrosing alveolitis
2. Sarcoid infiltration
3. Thoracic cage deformity
4. Pleural effusion
5. Pleural fibrosis
6. Dust diseases

OBSTRUCTIVE DEFECT (REDUCED FEV_1 >VC)

$$\frac{FEV_1}{FVC} = <70 \text{ per cent}$$

Causes
1. Chronic bronchitis
2. Asthma
3. Bronchiectasis and other residual inflammatory conditions

Figure 4.1 Spirometry. FVC = forced vital capacity, FEV_1 = forced expiratory volume in 1 second

Lung volumes

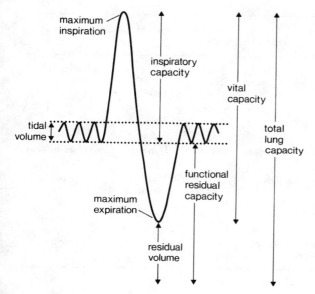

Figure 4.2 Lung volumes

Causes of a reduced vital capacity

1. Severe airways obstruction – the most common
2. Reduced lung volume
   i.   pulmonary oedema
   ii. collapsed lobes or lungs
   iii. large effusions
   iv. pulmonary fibrosis
   v.   diffuse infiltrations
3. Skeletal abnormality – kyphoscoliosis
4. Weak respiratory muscles – all infrequent
   i.   muscular dystrophies
   ii. myopathies
   iii. Guillain–Barré polyneuropathy
   iv. myasthenia gravis

Physical signs of common lung conditions

TABLE 4.1

	Effusion	Consolidation	Extensive collapse	Pneumothorax	Emphysema
Chest wall movement	↓ on affected side	Slightly ↓ over area	↓ over area	↓ over affected area	↓ bilaterally
Mediastinal shift	To opposite side	Nil	To affected side	To opposite side	Nil
Percussion note	Stony dull	Impaired	Impaired	Hyper-resonant	Hyper-resonant
Breath sounds	Diminished vesicular Bronchial at level of fluid	Bronchial	Diminished vesicular	May be absent	Diminished
Added sounds	Nil; at times a rub	Creps	Nil	Nil	Wheezing or nil

Respiratory failure

DEFINITION

If due to lung disease, the arterial Po_2 is <60 mmHg (8.0 kPa) in a patient breathing air at sea level, respiratory failure is present.
Type I – Po_2 reduced with a normal or low Pco_2 – <50 mmHg (6.7 kPa)
Type II – hypoxaemia with hypercapnia – Po_2 <60 mmHg (8 kPa) and Pco_2 >50 mmHg (6.7 kPa)

CAUSES OF TYPE I RESPIRATORY FAILURE

The most frequent event is an increased variability in ventilation/perfusion ($\dot{V}/\dot{Q}$) ratios. This group of diseases leads to perfused alveoli with little air so blood shunts without oxygenation.

1. Early chronic bronchitis
2. Acute asthma
3. Thromboembolism
4. Fibrosing alveolitis
5. Pneumonia and lobe collapse
6. Acute pulmonary oedema

CAUSES OF TYPE II RESPIRATORY FAILURE

The most common in clinical practice.

1. Later chronic bronchitis – acute exacerbation
2. Acute asthma
3. Narcotic overdose
4. Mechanical abnormalities of the thorax
    i. scoliosis
    ii. ankylosing spondylitis
5. Neuromuscular diseases
    i.   muscular dystrophy
    ii. myasthenia gravis
    iii. peripheral neuropathy
6. Primary alveolar hypoventilation

Transfer factor ($T_L CO$)

DEFINITION

The quantity of gas transferred in a given time as a result of a measured average tension gradient from alveoli to pulmonary capillary blood.
$T_L CO$ expressed as mmol/minute/mmHg (mmol.min^{-1}. kPa^{-1}) and carbon monoxide transfer coefficient (Kco) is the $T_L CO$ per litre of the volume of alveolar gas (VA).

CONDITIONS AFFECTING $T_L CO$

Lung disease

1. Asthma   Normal or ↑
2. Bronchitis   Normal or ↓
3. Emphysema   ↓
4. Diffuse infiltrations ↓
5. Pulmonary emboli   ↓
6. Ageing   ↓
7. Fresh lung bleeding   ↑

Heart disease

1. Pulmonary oedema   ↓
2. Low cardiac output ↓
3. Hyperkinetic states ↑
4. L to R shunts   ↑

Blood disease

1. Anaemia   ↓
2. Polycythaemia   ↑

Haemoptysis

  1. Bronchial carcinoma – spots of blood ⎫
  2. Tuberculosis ⎫   ⎬ the most
  3. Pulmonary infarct ⎬ 'pure blood'   ⎭ common causes
  4. Bronchiectasis ⎭
  5. Pneumonia – blood streaking of purulent sputum
  6. Foreign body
  7. Lung abscess
  8. Polyarteritis nodosa ⎫
  9. Mycoses ⎬ rare
10. Mitral stenosis
11. Pulmonary haemosiderosis ⎭
12. Remains unexplained in 30 per cent of patients

CXR findings in haemoptysis

  1. Normal – 50 per cent
  2. Carcinoma
  3. Collapse – carcinoma or foreign body
  4. Consolidation – endobronchial carcinoma
  5. Tuberculosis with or without cavitation
  6. Left ventricular failure
  7. Infection or infarction
  8. Cystic fibrosis
  9. Mycetoma
10. Wegener's granulomatosis

DIFFERENTIATION OF HAEMOPTYSIS FROM HAEMATEMESIS

1. History usually clarifies virtually all cases
2. Lung blood is usually bright red, has an alkaline pH and the sputum contains macrophages filled with haemosiderin
3. Gastric blood is dark, has an acid pH and may be contaminated by food particles

Clubbing

The loss of the acute angle between nail and nail bed. Best seen when the finger is viewed from the side. The nail bed may be fluctuant, with increased transverse nail curvature.

CAUSES
1. Lung cancer – easily the most common
2. Chronic suppurative infection
    i. abscess
    ii. bronchiectasis
    iii. cystic fibrosis
    iv. chronic empyema
    v. pulmonary tuberculosis
3. Fibrosing alveolitis
4. Mesothelioma
5. Cyanotic congenital heart disease
6. Cirrhosis
7. Inflammatory bowel disease
8. Familial and congenital

Pleural effusion

1. Increased capillary pressure – transudates; protein <30 g/ℓ
    i. heart failure – common
    ii. fluid overload
    iii. hypoprotinaemia

2. Increased capillary permeability – exudates: protein >30 g/ℓ
    i. bronchial carcinoma involving pleura (primary or secondary) – often bloody and recurrent
    ii. pleural inflammation
        (a) pneumonia
        (b) tuberculosis
        (c) infarction – often bloody
        (d) mesothelioma
        (e) lymphoma and leukaemia
    iii. subdiaphragmatic disease
        (a) sub-phrenic abscess
        (b) acute pancreatitis – usually left-sided
        (c) chylothorax – rare

3. Left pleural effusion with surgical emphysema of chest wall – found after a ruptured oesophagus

Causes of slow resolution of a pneumonia

1. Obstruction to a bronchus – tumour or foreign body
2. Formation of an abscess or empyema
3. Recurrent aspiration from oesophagus
4. Incorrect antibiotic therapy
5. Impaired host resistance (*see* page 257)

Causes of lung cavities

1. Tuberculosis – typically upper lobe of one side and apical segment of lower lobe of the other
2. Cavitated squamous bronchial carcinoma
3. Other causes – *see* Lung Abscess below

} the most common

Causes of lung abscesses

1. Bronchial obstruction – tumour, foreign body
2. Infection
    i.   *Staphylococcus pyogenes*
    ii. *Klebsiella*
    iii. *Legionella pneumophila*
3. Aspiration pneumonia
    i.   oesophageal obstruction
    ii. drowning
    iii. coma
    iv. spill from an abscess
4. Pulmonary infarct which becomes infected
5. *Entomoeba histolytica*

Pneumothorax

1. Primary – young adult males chiefly; fairly common; benign (but frequently recur)
2. Secondary
    i.   chronic bronchitis – usually due to rupture of an emphysematous bulla
    ii.   pulmonary tuberculosis
    iii. asthma
    iv.   lung abscess
    v.   bronchial carcinoma
    vi.   pulmonary fibrosis
    vii. traumatic
    viii. catamenial (at the time of menstruation)

} infrequent

Pneumonic pathogens

BACTERIAL

1. *Streptococcus pneumoniae* – lobar pneumonia and chronic bronchitis

2. *Staphylococcus pyogenes*
3. *Haemophilus influenzae* – chronic bronchitis
4. *Streptococcus pyogenes*
5. *Pseudomonas aeruginosa* – usually acquired in hospital
6. *Klebsiella pneumoniae* – often cavitates
7. *Legionella pneumophila*
8. *Mycobacterium tuberculosis*

MYCOPLASMAL

Mycoplasma pneumoniae – commonest non-bacterial cause of pneumonia

VIRAL

1. Adenoviruses
2. Coxsackie and echovirus
3. Respiratory syncitial virus
4. Varicella
5. Infectious mononucleosis

the pneumonia may be primary or complicate an infection by one of these viruses. Clinically similar to mycoplasmal pneumonia

Determinants of postoperative pneumonias

1. Chronic respiratory disease
2. Chest and upper abdominal operations
3. Weight >120 kg
4. Smokers
5. Men > women
6. Operations lasting > 2 hours

Pneumonia and hepatitis

1. *Mycoplasma pneumoniae*
2. *Chlamydia psittaci*
3. *Coxiella burnetii*
4. *Legionella pneumophila*
5. Cytomegalovirus
6. Toxoplasmosis

Elevation of one dome of the diaphragm

Right dome is 1 to 2 cm higher than the left in all phases of respiration

1. Excessive gas in stomach
2. Basal pulmonary infection or infarction
3. Collapse of lower or middle lobe on the affected side

4. Spinal curvature
5. Phrenic nerve damage
   i.   malignant disease
   ii. trauma
   iii. neuropathy
6. Sub-phrenic abscess.

Chronic bronchitis and emphysema

DEFINITIONS

Chronic bronchitis
Clinically, an excess of mucus causing persisting cough and sputum for more than 3 months per year for 3 consecutive years. The principal disease of central airways.

Emphysema
Pathologically, dilatation of air spaces distal to terminal bronchioles with destruction of respiratory tissue and loss of elastic recoil. The FEV_1 may well be normal, but tests of small airway function produce abnormal results.

The two conditions overlap to a considerable extent in most patients. The common pathogens are *Haemophilus influenzae* and *Streptococcus pneumoniae*; they frequently are both present during an acute exacerbation.

CAUSAL AGENTS

1. Cigarette smoking
   (dose-dependent)   } shown to be causative in
2. Low social class   } epidemiological surveys
3. Atmospheric pollution   }
4. Recurrent respiratory infections
5. Possibly, alcohol abuse

HOST SUSCEPTIBILITY FACTORS

1. Cystic fibrosis   }
2. Immotile cilia syndrome   } not common
3. Severe α_1-antitrypsin deficiency }

Clinical patterns of chronic bronchitis

TABLE 4.2

Clinical pattern	'Blue bloater'	'Pink puffer'
Chest deformity	Moderate	Marked hyperinflation
Breathlessness	Moderate	Marked
Central cyanosis	Yes	No
Cor pulmonale	Yes	No
Arterial P_{O_2}	Reduced	} Relatively normal
Arterial P_{CO_2}	Raised	

While these two groups can be separated clinically many patients have features of both. The 'blue bloater' is more common.

Chest X-ray appearances

See page 56

1. Flattened low diaphragms
2. Long thin heart shadow
3. Horizontal pattern of ribs
4. Eleventh rib visible – due to low diaphragm
5. Reduction in distal vascular pattern – emphysema
6. Dilatation of the heart when in failure

Respiratory function tests

1. FEV_1 reduced
2. Obstructive pattern – FEV_1/FVC <70 per cent
3. Total lung capacity (TLC) increased – hyperinflation
4. Reduced vital capacity
5. Residual volume (RV) increased
6. RV/TLC > the normal – 30–35 per cent
7. $T_L co$ reduced

PROGNOSIS

30 per cent of patients survive beyond 5 years once cor pulmonale has developed.

Malignant disease of the lungs

1. Bronchial carcinoma – majority arise from central airways
     i.   squamous cell – cavitate   50 per cent
    ii.   small (oat) cell – invade rapidly   20 per cent
   iii.   adenocarcinoma – lung periphery   20 per cent
    iv.   large cell   10 per cent

2. Secondary metastases – often multiple (*see* page 133)
3. Bronchial adenomas – present earlier than carcinoma
4. Infiltration by Hodgkin's or lymphosarcoma
5. Carcinoid ⎫
6. Cylindromata ⎬ rare

Clinical features of bronchial carcinoma

1. Local (primary) symptoms
2. Metastatic – within and outside the lung
3. Male to female ratio now 2:1
4. Non-metastatic extrapulmonary features

LOCAL SYMPTOMS

1. Cough	80 per cent	
2. Haemoptysis	70 per cent	
3. Dyspnoea	60 per cent	of patients
4. Chest pain over site of lesion	40 per cent	
5. Wheeze	15 per cent	

INTRATHORACIC SPREAD

Present in up to 70 per cent of patients at presentation. Bronchial carcinomas metastasize widely

1. Pleural effusion – exudate, bloody, recurrent
2. Recurrent laryngeal paralysis – hoarse with bovine cough
3. Phrenic paralysis – raised diaphragm
4. Horner's syndrome – sympathetic ganglia; *see* page 228
5. Brachial plexus involvement – Pancoast syndrome – T1
6. Chest wall invasion – direct or from a metastatic deposit
7. Pericarditis – involvement of pericardium
8. Superior vena caval obstruction – right paratracheal nodes

EXTRATHORACIC SPREAD

1. Metastasis to
    i.   brain
    ii. bone – chiefly ribs, vertebrae, femora or humeri
    iii. liver ⎫
    iv. suprarenals ⎬ usually asymptomatic
    v.   neck nodes
2. Weight loss, anorexia and malaise. An associated poor prognosis

NON-METASTATIC FEATURES

1. Endocrine – all infrequent
   i. SIADH *see* page 68; chiefly oat cell tumours
   ii. hypercalcaemia – chiefly squamous cell
   iii. ectopic ACTH – usually oat cell tumours
2. Skeleton
   i. clubbing – in 50 per cent of squamous tumours
   ii. hypertrophic pulmonary osteoarthropathy
3. Vascular
   i. bleeding disorders
   ii. thrombophlebitis migrans – the least common
   iii. non-bacterial endocarditis
4. Neuromyopathies – all rare
   i. neuropathy
   ii. proximal myopathy
   iii. cerebellar degeneration
   iv. myasthenia
   v. dermatomyositis

Circumscribed lesions ('coin lesions')

Vaguely circular chest X-ray opacity with clear surrounding lung.
May be found at any site. Size – few mm – 10 cm.

COMMON

1. Bronchial carcinoma – spicular outline: cavitation
2. Metastasis, single or multiple
3. Tuberculosis – usually upper lobes with satellite lesions: may calcify
4. Hydatid cyst ⎫
5. Histoplasmoma – may calcify ⎬ endemic areas

RARE

6. Rheumatoid nodule – may cavitate
7. Infarct – may cavitate
8. Bronchial adenoma
9. Hamartoma – calcified
10. A–V fistula
11. PMF
12. Wegener's granulomatosis
13. Lipid pneumonia

Causes of a chronic cough

DEFINITION

Troublesome cough lasting more than 3 weeks. Chiefly due to mechanical or chemical stimulation of larynx, carina, trachea or main bronchi.

1. Lung
    i. chronic bronchitis
    ii. asthma
    iii. carcinoma
    iv. left ventricular failure
    v. tuberculosis
    vi. sarcoid
    vii. fungal infections

2. Extrapulmonary
    i. postnasal drip
    ii. gastro-oesophageal reflux

3. Extrathoracic
    i. subphrenic abscess
    ii. irritation of external auditory meatus
    iii. habit cough – diagnosis of exclusion

Indications for steroids in sarcoidosis

1. Hypercalcaemia – occurs in about 6–10 per cent of cases
2. Rapidly progressive lung disease
3. Ocular ⎱
4. Brain   ⎰ involvement
5. Myocardial ⎰
6. Disfiguring skin lesions

Causes of raised serum angiotensin converting enzyme activity

1. Active sarcoid
2. Tuberculosis
3. Asbestosis
4. Berylliosis and silicosis
5. Gaucher's disease

Adult respiratory distress syndrome (ARDS)

Acute progressive respiratory failure with serious underlying disease or trauma usually without previous lung disease or direct pulmonary damage. Bilateral diffuse infiltrate seen on chest X-ray without cardiomegaly or venous congestion. Severe hypoxaemia with shunting, stiff lungs and reduced lung volumes increasing work of breathing. Alveoli fill with protein-rich fluid from lung capillaries. Pao_2 reduced and difficult to control despite increasing the fraction of oxygen in inspired air (F_1o_2). Thus alveolar–arterial oxygen tension difference widens with increased venous admixture or right to left shunting. Pao_2 often as low as 30–40 mmHg (4.0–5.3 kPa) despite F_1o_2 of 40–60% or more. Mortality 50–60% or greater if other major organ failure. Full recovery possible.

CAUSES

1. Trauma, not necessarily thoracic; burns
2. Gram-negative septicaemias
3. Acute pancreatitis, DIC, air or amniotic fluid embolism
4. Chemical pneumonitis
    i.   inhalation of gastric acid
    ii. near drowning
    iii. smoke or chemical irritants
    iv. paraquat

Bronchoscopy

INDICATIONS

1. Abnormal chest X-ray with
    i.   one or more persistent opacities
    ii. persistent shadowing
2. Normal chest X-ray with
    i.   haemoptysis
    ii. positive sputum cytology
3. Removal of foreign bodies
4. Excessive secretions
5. Opportunist infections

CONTRA-INDICATIONS

1. Inadequate ventilatory reserve
2. Severe asthma
3. Copious haemoptysis
4. SVC obstruction
5. Open TB

Lung features of connective tissue diseases

1. Rheumatoid disease
   i.   pleural effusions – low glucose concentration
   ii. fibrosing alveolitis – occasionally
   iii. nodules – rare
   iv. Caplan's syndrome – RA, nodules in dust-exposed workers
   v.   Obstructive bronchitis and bronchiolitis
2. SLE
   i.   secondary infection
   ii. pleurisy
   iii. pneumonitis
   iv. fibrosing alveolitis – rare
3. Polyarteritis nodosa
   i.   asthma with eosinophilia
   ii. haemoptysis
4. Wegener's granulomatosis
   i.   nodules
   ii. haemoptysis

   } rare diseases

5. Progressive systemic sclerosis – scleroderma
   i.   interstitial fibrosis
   ii. aspiration pneumonia

Diffuse pulmonary fibrosis

1. Pneumoconiosis – inorganic or organic dusts
2. Granulomatous diseases – TB, sarcoid
3. Drug-induced – nitrofurantoin, busulphan
4. Chronic pulmonary oedema
5. Collagen diseases – RA, PSS, Sjögren's disease
6. X-irradiation
7. Lymphangitis carcinomatosa

   } fibrosis in these conditions is a complication of the original disease

8. Cryptogenic fibrosing alveolitis – rare; unknown aetiology
9. Extrinsic allergic alveolitis – Type III reaction
   i.   farmer's lung-antigen *Micropolyspora faeni*
   ii. bird-fancier's lung – antigen: avian serum protein

   } no idiopathic or allergic diseases

Occupational lung disease

Nearly all are avoidable.

MINERAL DUSTS: COAL, SILICATES, IRON, TIN, ALUMINIUM, TUNGSTEN

1. Pneumoconiosis
   i.   simple – multiple discrete opacities, without functional impairment
   ii. complicated – progressive (PMF) nodular lesions
   iii. Caplan's syndrome – in coal workers with RA
2. Asbestosis
   i.   pleural plaques
   ii. fibrosis
   iii. mesothelioma
   iv. bronchial carcinoma
3. Silicosis – progressive, eggshell calcification of hilar nodes

CHRONIC BRONCHITIS

Heavy industry with polluted atmospheres

ORGANIC DUSTS

1. Farmer's lung – *Micropolyspora faeni* and *Thermophilia vulgaris*
2. Bagassosis – contaminated sugar cane
3. Mushroom-worker's lung
4. Byssinosis

OCCUPATIONAL LUNG CANCER

1. Asbestos workers
2. Nickel-refining
3. Chromate workers
4. Retort house workers – gas works

OCCUPATIONAL ASTHMA

Variable airflow obstruction caused by specific exposure at work. Very many causes recognized including

1. Organic dusts – (*see* above)
2. Flux used in soldering
3. Red cedar wood
4. Washing powder manufacture
5. Some drug manufacture
6. Plastic foams in furniture making
7. Epoxy resins

FEV_1 normal between attacks, symptoms improve at weekends. FEV_1 or PFR have to be recorded at work

Pulmonary eosinophilia

An excess of eosinophils in sputum and peripheral blood (>6 per cent)

1. Asthmatic pulmonary eosinophilia due to allergic bronchopulmonary aspergillosis
2. Simple – Loeffler's syndrome; short duration illness associated with *Ascaris, Ankylostoma* or *Trichuris*
3. Prolonged – unknown cause
4. Tropical – due to filarial infestation, Ascaris or Schistosoma
5. Drug reactions
   i.   methotrexate
   ii. busulphan
   iii. nitrofurantoin
6. Collagen vascular disease – polyarteritis nodosa, Churg–Strauss syndrome

Pneumonic conditions in compromised hosts

Immune-compromised hosts comprise one of the three different categories of patients

1. Those with myeloma, leukaemia or lymphorecticular neoplasms – *see* pages 124–129
2. Those receiving steroids or cytotoxic drugs, or both. Groups 1 and 2 tend to overlap
3. Those with primary immune deficiency diseases – page 257, including acquired immune deficiency syndrome (AIDS)

These patients are prone to infections due to

1. *Mycobacterium tuberculosis*
2. Pseudomonas, Klebsiellae or *E. coli*
3. Herpes simplex, cytomegalovirus or varicella-zoster viruses
4. *Pneumocystis carinii* – particularly in AIDS patients
5. *Candida albicans*
6. *Cryptococcus neoformans*
7. *Aspergillus fumigatus*
8. *Strongyloides stercoralis*

They may also suffer lung damage from

1. Direct toxicity from the drugs busulphan or bleomycin
2. X-irradiation
3. Extension of tumour into the lung – *see* page 44
4. Bleeding into the lung from thrombocytopenia as a result of
   i. the primary disease – leukaemias
   ii. the cytotoxic therapy

Mediastinal masses

ANTERIOR

1. Thymoma
2. Dermoid cysts
3. Teratomas
4. Goitres – ^{131}I scan

MIDDLE

1. Hiatus hernia – Ba swallow
2. Pleuropericardial cysts
3. Bronchogenic cysts

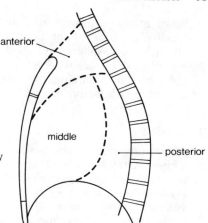

POSTERIOR

1. Aortic aneurysms – usually descending
2. Paravertebral abscess – usually tuberculous
3. Neurogenic tumours – all rare
   i.   neurilemmoma
   ii. neurofibroma
   iii. ganglioneuroma
   iv. neuroblastoma

Causes of hilar and mediastinal lymphadenopathy

1. Metastatic carcinoma
   i. almost always bronchial primarily
   ii. occasionally primary in breast or colon
2. Lymphoma
   asymmetrical and often symptomatic
3. Hodgkin's disease
   i. nodes may be huge
   ii. anterior mediastinum may be involved
4. Sarcoid
   symmetrical, bilateral, asymptomatic
5. Tuberculosis
   i.   usually asymmetrical
   ii. primary infection in children often symptomatic
   iii. common in Asians and others who emigrate to Western
        countries

Lung scanning

TECHNIQUE AND MATERIALS

1. Perfusion ($\dot{Q}$ scans) – to demonstrate regional distribution of
   lung blood flow by scanning or 'imaging' (gamma camera) the

lungs after an intravenous dose of labelled particles which localize in some of the pulmonary capillaries. ^{99m}Tc labelled albumin microspheres are used

2. Ventilation ($\dot{V}$ scans) – to demonstrate distribution of gas to the lungs by scanning the lungs after the inspiration of an insoluble radioactive gas such as xenon–133

APPLICATIONS

1. Pulmonary embolism – this lesion may not be demonstrable on a chest X-ray but a $\dot{V}/\dot{Q}$ scan will demonstrate normal ventilation with impaired perfusion of the infarcted area
2. Airways obstruction – patchy areas of abnormal perfusion and ventilation match each other
3. Lung cancer – there may be minor defects in ventilation but large loss of perfusion due to pulmonary vessel involvement
4. Heart disease – chiefly used to assess pulmonary venous hypertension caused by LVF or mitral stenosis or in recurrent pulmonary thromboembolism. The normal basal predominance of perfusion is lost or reversed. The upper lobe diversion provides a guide to left atrial pressure. Sequential studies may be used to assess treatment

Indications for thoracic CT scanning

MEDIASTINUM

1. To define a known mass
2. To differentiate between fat, vessels or nodes
3. To investigate occult mediastinal disease
4. To examine the great vessels and congenital heart abnormalities

LUNGS

1. Metastasis
   i.   pre-operatively
   ii. to define apparently solitary lesions
   iii. to assess success of chemotherapy
2. Assessment of early parenchymal disease or bullae

Chapter 5

Chest radiographs

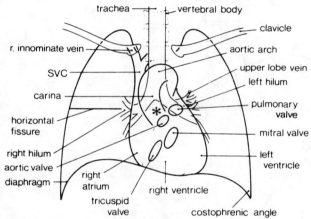

Figure 5.1a Features recognizable on a postero-anterior chest X-ray. Full inspiration is judged by being able to see below the border of the right twelfth rib. The asterisk indicates the position of the left atrium within the heart shadow under the carina. The position of the heart valves are shown although the valves are not seen on a chest X-ray

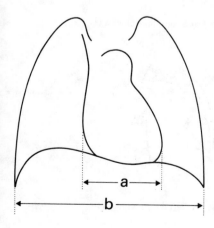

Figure 5.1b The cardiothoracic ratio = a/b. In health it is <45 per cent

53

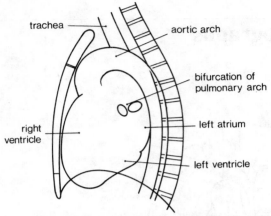

Figure 5.2 Features recognizable on a left lateral chest X-ray

Lobar collapse

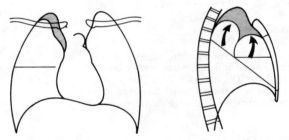

Figure 5.3 Right upper lobe collapse; PA and right lateral views

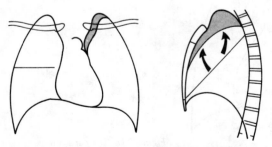

Figure 5.4 Left upper lobe collapse; PA and left lateral views

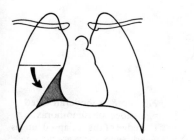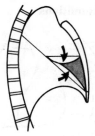

Figure 5.5 Middle lobe collapse; PA and right lateral views

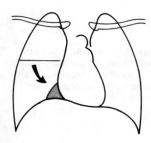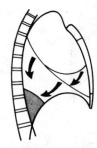

Figure 5.6 Right lower lobe collapse; PA and right lateral views

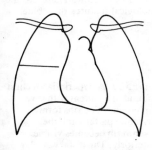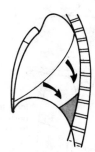

Figure 5.7 Left lower lobe collapse; PA and left lateral
views. The left lower lobe is 'hidden' behind the heart

Other pulmonary conditions

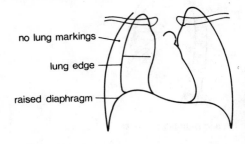

no lung markings

lung edge

raised diaphragm

Figure 5.8 A moderate-sized right-sided pneumothorax. The edge of the collapsed lung is clearly seen; there are no lung markings beyond it

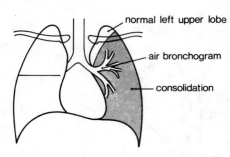

normal left upper lobe

air bronchogram

consolidation

Figure 5.9 Consolidation of the whole of the left lower lobe. There is no loss of lung volume; an 'air bronchogram' is present. The trachea is central

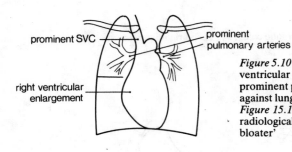

prominent SVC

prominent pulmonary arteries

right ventricular enlargement

Figure 5.10 Cor pulmonale. Right ventricular enlargement and prominent pulmonary arteries set against lung changes shown in *Figure 15.11* below. These are the radiological features of a 'blue bloater'

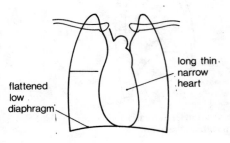

long thin narrow heart

flattened low diaphragm

Figure 5.11 A hyperinflated chest as found in a patient with severe emphysema. The ribs form a horizontal pattern and the eleventh rib becomes visible posteriorly. The distal vascular pattern in the lungs is lost. This appearance is found in the 'pink puffer'

Pulmonary sarcoid

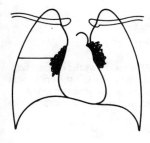

Figure 5.12 Stage I – Bilateral hilar adenopathy without lung involvement. Two-thirds of cases regress permanently after this stage

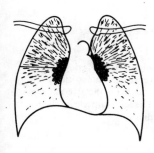

Figure 5.13 Stage II – Hilar adenopathy with lung opacities most marked in mid and upper zones. Lung abnormalities may develop as adenopathy regresses. Resolution occurs in one-third of cases

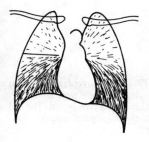

Figure 5.14 Stage III – Pulmonary fibrosis. No adenopathy. Irreversible disease; death will occur from respiratory failure. These features develop in about 5 per cent of patients with lung sarcoid

Radiology of left ventricular failure

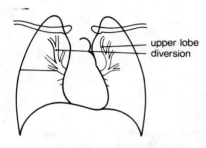

Figure 5.15 This shows the earliest sign of a failing left ventricle – the prominent upper zone veins due to diversion of blood from the lower oedematous zones

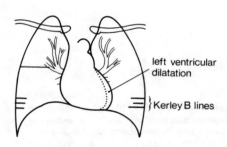

Figure 5.16 Kerley B lines represent interstitial oedema in the alveolar septa. The left ventricle has begun to dilate

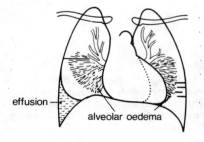

Figure 5.17 Diffuse alveolar oedema in a butterfly wing pattern is present. A pleural effusion has developed. The patient would usually be critically ill at this stage

Some characteristic cardiac X-rays

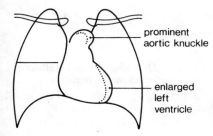

prominent
aortic knuckle

enlarged
left
ventricle

Figure 5.18 Moderate left ventricular
hypertrophy as may occur in established
hypertension. The ascending aorta is
slightly enlarged

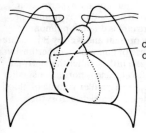

distorted dilated
descending aorta

Figure 5.19 Severe left ventricular
hypertrophy with aneurysmal dilatation
of the thoracic aorta

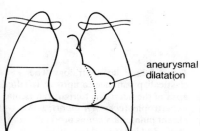

aneurysmal
dilatation

Figure 5.20 A large left ventricular
aneurysm. The left border of the heart is
distorted by a rounded shadow with
characteristic tip-tilting

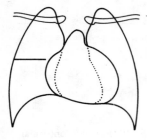

Figure 5.21 A large pericardial effusion. No specific aetiology is implied

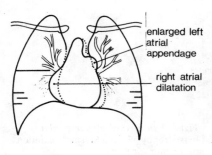

enlarged left atrial appendage

right atrial dilatation

Figure 5.22 Fully established mitral stenosis with pulmonary hypertension. The left atrial appendage is prominent, the right atrium is dilated, pulmonary plethora is present and Kerley B lines are seen because of pulmonary hypertension. The aorta is a little smaller than normal and the left ventricle is normal or smaller in size because a smaller volume of blood reaches the left ventricle across the stenotic valve

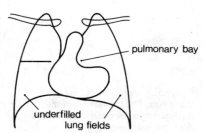

pulmonary bay

underfilled lung fields

Figure 5.23 Fallot's tetralogy. The classical appearance comprises: 1. Tilted apex of the heart due to right ventricular hypertrophy (*coeur-en-sabot*); 2. An absent pulmonary conus producing a 'bay'; 3. Underfilled lung fields

Chapter 6

Metabolic and electrolyte disorders

Acid–base disturbances

Acidosis
When arterial pH is below the normal range of 7.36–7.42 or would be if compensatory mechanisms were inoperative.

Alkalosis
When arterial pH is above the normal range or would be if compensatory mechanisms fail.

Respiratory disturbances
All related to altered elimination of CO_2

Metabolic or non-respiratory disturbances
Presence of excessive quantities of acid or alkali, endogenous or exogenous.

Henderson–Hasselbalch equation
The relationship of arterial pH to $PaCO_2$ and bicarbonate:

$$pH = 6.1 + \log_{10} \frac{[HCO_3^-]}{(0.03 \times Paco_2)}$$

when $Paco_2$ is expressed in mmHg. If kPa units are used 0.225 must replace 0.03.

'Standard bicarbonate'
What the bicarbonate would have been if the blood had been incubated *in vitro* at a $Paco_2$ of 40 mmHg (5.33 kPa).

'Base deficit or excess'
The amount of alkali or acid required to titrate *in vitro* 1ℓ of blood to pH 7.4 at 40 mmHg.

Anion gap
$(Na^+ + K^+) - (Cl^- + HCO_3^-)$. Normally about 10–18. Metabolic acidoses with a normal anion gap are due to loss of bicarbonate with replacement by chloride; those with a high gap, bicarbonate has been titrated by acids, endogenous or exogenous, without altering the concentration of the plasma chloride.

61 .

Respiratory acid–base disturbances

RESPIRATORY ACIDOSES

pH $\downarrow$ P_{CO_2} $\uparrow$

1. Lung disease
   i. chronic obstructive airways disease
   ii. severe asthma
   iii. large airway obstruction
2. Respiratory centre disease – depressant drugs; opiates, anaesthetics, barbiturates, dextropropoxyphene
3. Neuromuscular and skeletal disease
   i. flail chest
   ii. restriction – ankylosing spondylitis, bad kyphoscoliosis, gross obesity
   iii. muscular weakness – muscular dystrophy, myasthenia gravis, ascending Guillain–Barré, motor neuron disease

RESPIRATORY ALKALOSES

Hyperventilation; pH $\uparrow$ P_{CO_2} $\downarrow$

1. Pulmonary embolism, collapse, pneumothorax
2. Stimulation to respiratory centre
   i. via chemoreceptors
      (a) low inspired oxygen concentration
      (b) alveolar-capillary diffusion block
      (c) R to L shunts
      (d) CO poisoning
   ii. salicylate poisoning – early stages
   iii. damage to respiratory centre
3. Psychological – hysteria or anxiety

METABOLIC ACIDOSIS

pH $\downarrow$ P_{CO_2} $\downarrow$

1. Ketoacidosis – diabetic, starvation
2. Lactic acidosis Type A ⎱ *see* pages 63–4
3. Lactic acidosis Type B ⎰
4. Advanced chronic renal failure; later phases of salicylate poisoning

⎫
⎬ raised anion
⎭ gap; e.g.
   excess acids

5. Bicarbonate loss
   i. diarrhoea
   ii. small gut, biliary or pancreatic fistulae
6. Renal tubular acidosis
7. Ammonium chloride load

} normal anion gap; e.g. bicarbonate loss with chloride replacement

METABOLIC ALKALOSES

pH ↑ PCO_2 ↑

1. Excess alkali
   i. forced alkaline diuresis
   ii. excessive bicarbonate treatment of metabolic acidosis
   iii. excess alkali in chronic renal failure
2. Excess acid loss
   i. potassium depletion ⎫
   ii. hyperaldosteronism ⎬ renal loss   *predominal aiduria*
   iii. chloride depletion ⎭
   iv. pyloric stenosis – gastric and renal loss

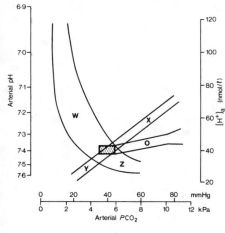

Figure 6.1 An acid–base diagram.
W = metabolic acidosis;
X = acute respiratory acidosis;
O = chronic respiratory acidosis;
Y = acute respiratory alkalosis;
Z = metabolic alkalosis

Lactic acidosis

Normal resting plasma lactate is usually <1 mmol/ℓ. Clinically important concentrations are 15 mmol/ℓ or more.

1. Type A – primary circulatory failure or severe hypoxia
   i. shock
   ii. hypotension
   iii. hypoxia

2. Type B – no primary circulatory failure ·
   i. biguanide therapy
   ii. fructose or sorbitol infused too rapidly
   iii. ethanol or methanol poisoning
   iv. acute liver failure

Water metabolism

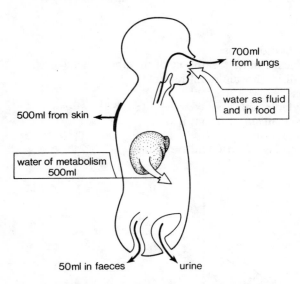

500ml from skin

700ml from lungs

water as fluid and in food

water of metabolism 500ml

50ml in faeces

urine

Figure 6.2 Water balance in an adult in a temperate climate

Body fluid compartments

Intravascular space   5 ℓ } extracellular } in a
Interstitial space   14 ℓ } space   } 70 kg
Intracellular space   23 ℓ   } man

Water excess

Occurs when an excess of water is taken or given proportionate to
the ability to excrete. Main symptoms are related to excess fluid in
the brain – from headaches to coma. Oedema is not a feature of
water excess alone. The serum osmolarity – normal 280–295

mmol/ℓ – and the plasma sodium concentration fall in the absence of sodium depletion.

CAUSES

1. Excess i.v. fluids especially post-operatively – common
2. Acute oliguric renal failure
3. Advanced chronic renal failure
4. Inappropriate ADH secretion – *see* page 68
5. Compulsive water drinking ⎫
6. Glucocorticoid deficiency ⎬ rare
7. Hypothalamic lesions ⎭

Water deficiency

Chief symptom is thirst; fall in blood pressure is a late sign. Serum osmolarity and plasma sodium rise.

CAUSES

1. No water available
2. Patient too ill to drink
3. Osmotic diuresis
   i. diabetic coma
   ii. non-ketotic hyperosmolar coma
4. Diabetes insipidus – rare
   i. cranial
   ii. nephrogenic

Sodium excess

Sodium excess is usually accompanied by an equivalent retention of water and chloride.

CAUSES

1. Excessive NaCl especially post-operatively
2. Heart failure – although the primary disorder is impaired ventricular function
3. Hypoalbuminaemic conditions – *see* page 70; secondary hyper-aldosteronism
4. Chronic renal failure – late phases
5. Primary hyperaldosteronism – rare

Sodium deficiency

Usually accompanied by approximately equivalent deficits in water and chloride.

CAUSES

1. Excessive sweating
2. Gut loss
   i.   severe diarrhoea
   ii. fistulae
3. Renal losses
   i.   diabetes mellitus – osmotic diuresis
   ii. excessive diuretic therapy
   iii. renal salt wasting – conditions affecting the distal tubules and impairing their sodium conserving ability

Causes of hyperkalaemia

Normal potassium concentration 3.5–5.5 mmol/ℓ (mEq/ℓ)

1. Acute renal failure   } inability of adequate renal
2. Advanced chronic renal failure   } excretion
3. Potassium sparing agents –   } if given in the presence of poor
   amiloride, triamterene   } renal function
4. Spironolactone
5. Metabolic or respiratory acidosis

Causes of hypokalaemia

RENAL CAUSES

The main causes
1. Thiazide and loop diuretics   }
2. Diabetic ketoacidosis   } the most
3. Intravenous fluid therapy with   } common causes
   inadequate potassium supplements   }
4. Carbenoxolone or excess liquorice
5. Metabolic or respiratory alkalosis
6. Excess endogenous cortisol   }
7. Hyperaldosteronism   }
   i.   primary   }
   ii. secondary   } rare causes
        (a) accelerated hypertension   }
        (b) renal artery stenosis   }
8. Renal tubular acidosis   }

See also causes of hypokalaemia in the presence of renal failure – page 86.

GASTRO-INTESTINAL CAUSES

1. Any prolonged severe diarrhoea
2. Laxative abuse – usually women
3. Prolonged vomiting ⎫
4. Ureterosigmoid anastomosis ⎬ infrequent causes
5. Colonic mucus secreting neoplasms ⎭

Causes of hypokalaemic alkalosis

Plasma potassium <3.0 mmol/ℓ (mEq/ℓ), bicarbonate >30 mmol/ℓ (mEq/ℓ).

1. Diuretics – easily the most common
2. Hyperaldosteronism
    i. Primary (Conn's syndrome) – very rare
    ii. Secondary
        (a) pregnancy
        (b) congestive heart failure
        (c) vasodilator therapy
        (d) cirrhosis
        (e) nephrotic syndrome
        (f) purgatives
        (g) liquorice ⎫ high
        (h) carbenoxolone ⎭ dose

Severe hypophosphataemia

Serum phosphate <0.4 mmol/ℓ (<1.2 mg/100 ml)

1. During treatment of diabetic ketoacidosis
2. Following ethanol withdrawal in alcoholics
3. In total parenteral nutrition without phosphate supplements
4. Recovery after severe burns
5. Protein calorie malnutrition
6. Post-haemodialysis
7. Excess of phosphate binders

Moderate hypophosphataemia found in

1. Blood taken after venous stasis
2. Primary hyperparathyroidism

Causes of hyperphosphataemia

Serum phosphate >4.0 mmol/ℓ (>12.5 mg/100 ml)

1. Chronic renal failure
2. Hypoparathyroidism

Syndrome of inappropriate ADH secretion (SIADH)

FEATURES

1. Excessive water retention without oedema
2. Hyponatraemia
3. Urine sodium inappropriately high at >50 mmol/day
4. Low serum osmolarity <270 mmol/ℓ; urine osmolarity higher than that appropriate to the serum – 350–400 mmol/ℓ
5. Inability to excrete a water load
6. Symptoms develop when plasma sodium falls below 120–125 mmol/ℓ – nausea, debility, confusion, irritability, drowsiness, fits and coma

CAUSES

1. Ectopic ADH production
    i.   oat cell lung cancer – the most common; 40 per cent of cases
    ii. pulmonary tuberculosis
2. Excessive pituitary ADH
    i.   lung infections
    ii. positive pressure ventilation
    iii. cerebral trauma, infection, neoplasm, or haemorrhage
    iv. congestive cardiac failure
    v.   hypothyroidism
3. Drug associated
    i.   chlorpropamide
    ii. tricyclic antidepressants
    iii. thiazides
    iv. vincristine

Causes of hypercalcaemia

Serum Ca^{2+} > 2.6 mmol/ℓ (>10.5 mg/100 ml)

1. Malignancy associated
    i.   bony metastases – breast, bronchus, kidney, lymphoma
    ii. multiple myeloma – about 30 per cent of patients
    iii. ectopic PTH – *see* page 182

2. Hyperparathyroidism – *see* page 177
    i.   primary – often with mild hyperchloraemic acidosis
    ii. secondary – serum calcium is usually low
    iii. tertiary
3. Excess vitamin D or synthetic analogues – usually iatrogenic
4. Sarcoid – serum phosphate usually normal; calcium supressed with steroids
5. Late diuretic phase of acute renal failure
6. Hyperthyroidism
7. Idiopathic infantile – characteristic facies and supravalvular aortic stenosis
8. Milk-alkali syndrome
9. Cushing's disease and acromegaly
10. Lithium and thiazide therapy
11. Pluriglandular syndrome – *see* page 182

(items 5–11) } rare

Causes of hypercalciuria

24-hour urine Ca^{2+} > 7.5 mmol (>300 mg). May rise as high as 15.0 mmol (600 mg)/24 hours.

1. All causes of hypercalcaemia provided GFR > 30 ml/minute
2. Idiopathic hypercalciuria
3. Prolonged recumbency

Causes of hypocalcaemia

Serum Ca^{2+} < 2.25 mmol/ℓ (8.0 mg/100 ml).

1. Hypoparathyroidism
    i.   post-parathyroid surgery
    ii. post-thyroid surgery } usually transient
    iii. idiopathic – infrequent
2. Advanced (acidotic) chronic renal failure – Ca^{2+} about 2.0 mmol/ℓ; 8 mg/100 ml
3. Hypoalbuminaemia – diminished calcium binding sites
4. Severe prolonged vitamin D deficiency
5. Malnutrition } often related
6. Acute pancreatitis – transient hypocalcaemia in about 50 per cent
7. Neonatal hypocalcaemia – transient

Causes of hypocalciuria

24-hour urine Ca^{2+} < 2.5 mmol (100 mg)

1. All causes of hypocalcaemia
2. Acute nephrotic syndrome
3. CRF with GFR <25 ml/min

Causes of hypoalbuminaemia

Serum albumin <25 g/ℓ (2.5 g/100 ml)

1. Severe malnutrition ⎱ probably the most common causes
2. Severe malabsorption ⎰ worldwide. Infrequent in W. Europe
3. Catabolism of albumin as in severe infections
4. Advanced cirrhosis including frequent tapping of ascites
5. Following bleeding – dilutional
6. Severe diarrhoea as in ulcerative colitis
7. Nephrotic syndrome
8. Burns – loss of protein across raw areas

Causes of raised creatine kinase (CPK)

1. Myocardial infarction
2. Muscle injury
    i.   trauma
    ii. surgery
    iii. injections
    iv. severe exercise and post-seizures
3. Hypothyroidism
4. Alcoholic myopathy
5. Muscular dystrophies
6. Polymyositis

Causes of raised alkaline phosphatase

1. Growing children – 2–3 times greater than adult normal concentration
2. Liver disease (especially biliary obstruction)
    i.   obstructive jaundice
    ii. hepatitis
    iii. cirrhosis
3. Bone disease
    i.   secondary carcinoma
    ii. Paget's disease – elderly population
    iii. osteomalacia or rickets – see page 76
    iv. all types of hyperparathyroidism with bone disease
4. Pregnancy – may be raised in third trimester (from placenta)
5. Ectopic production by tumours (especially bronchus)

Causes of raised acid phosphatase

1. Metastasized carcinoma of prostate
   i. without metastases (25 per cent)
   ii. with skeletal metastases (80 per cent)
2. Following prostatic palpation (debated) or passage of a urinary catheter
3. Paget's disease of bone ⎫
4. Thrombocythaemia   ⎬ very occasionally

Causes of raised serum amylase

1. Acute pancreatitis – much raised
2. Severe diabetic ketoacidosis
3. Many acute abdominal surgical conditions
4. Mumps and manipulation of the parotids
5. Morphine administration
6. Tubal pregnancy

Causes of raised concentrations of aspartate aminotransferase (AST; SGOT)

1. Myocardial infarction ⎫
2. Acute liver diseases   ⎬ much increased
3. Congestive heart failure ⎫
4. Cardiac arrhythmias   ⎬ hepatic congestion
5. Obstructive jaundice   ⎫
6. Cirrhosis   ⎬ moderately increased
7. Damaged skeletal muscle ⎭
8. Severe haemolytic anaemias
9. Acute systemic infections, 'shock' with circulatory collapse
10. Acute pancreatitis
11. Pulmonary infarction

Raised enzymes after myocardial infarction

TABLE 6.1

Enzyme	Time after infarction		
	First rise (hours)	Peak (hours)	Duration (days)
Creatine kinase	6	24–48	3–4
Aspartate aminotransferase	6–8	24–48	4–5
Lactate dehydrogenase	12–24	48–72	7–12

Note that: CK also elevated in muscle disease and intramuscular injections
AST raised in liver and muscle disease
LDH activity raised in many conditions and in haemolysed blood

Porphyria

Porphyrias involve the biosynthetic pathway of haem. Porphobilinogen (PBG) is formed from 5-aminolaevulinate (ALA). There is a negative feedback from haem synthesis controlling ALA synthetase. The porphyrias are a group of conditions each of which results from an inborn error of one of the enzymes involved in haem synthesis, except for porphyria cutanea tarda symptomatica which is acquired but only in those who are genetically predisposed.

HEPATIC (normal red cell porphyrins)

All are autosomal dominants; may be precipitated by barbiturates, alcohol, fasting or infections.

	Acute attacks	Skin features
1. Acute intermittent – dark urine which fluoresces under u.v. light. Abdominal pain, neurological features, urinary ALA and PBG increased	+	–
2. Variegate – occurs in the Dutch in Cape Town	+	+ (50%)
3. Hereditary coproporphyria – very rare	+	+ (20%)
4. Secondary coproporphyria – alcoholism, lead poisoning, iron deficiency	+	+
5. Cutanea tarda symptomatica – commonest in UK	–	+

ERYTHROPOIETIC (increased red cell porphyrins)

1. Congenital – very rare, autosomal recessive	–	+
2. Protoporphyria – less rare, liver involvement in some, autosomal dominant	–	+

Hyperlipidaemias

There are four main lipoprotein classes found in serum

1. Chylomicrons – transport of dietary fat
2. Very low density lipoprotein (VLDL) – transport of endogenous triglyceride
3. Low density lipoproteins (LDL) – transport of cholesterol to peripheral cells
4. High density lipoproteins (HDL) – transport of cholesterol from peripheral cells

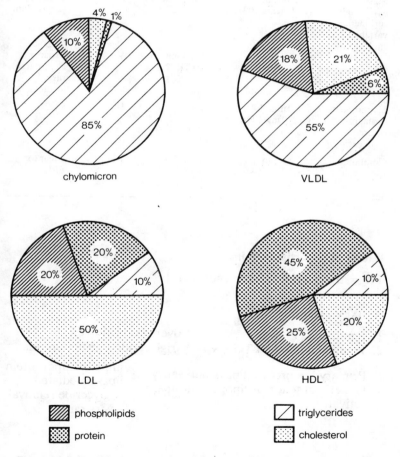

Figure 6.3 Schematic representation of the composition of the chief lipoproteins

Classification of hyperlipidaemia

TABLE 6.2

Class	Lipid concentrations	Lipoprotein abnormality	Fredrickson type	Stored serum
Hypertrigly-ceridaemia (with normal cholesterol)	1.8–12.0 mmol/ℓ (160–1050 mg/100 ml)	VLDL ↑	IV	Uniformly turbid
Massive hypertrigly-ceridaemia – variable cholesterol	>12.00 mmol/ℓ (>1050 mg/100 ml)	Chylomicrons	I	Creamy supernatant
		Chylomicrons+ VLDL ↑	V	Creamy supernatant, turbid intranatant
Hypercholest-erolaemia – normal triglyceride	>7.0 mmol/ℓ (>270 mg/100 ml)	LDL	IIa	Clear
Combined hyperlipid-aemia	>1.8 mmol/ℓ (>160 mg/100 ml)	LDL ↑ + VLDL ↑ β-VLDL	IIb III	Clear to turbid

Causes of hyperlipidaemia

TG = triglyceride, CH = cholesterol

PRIMARY – all rare

1. Familial TG
2. Familial combined TG + CH } over-production of triglyceride-rich lipoproteins

3. Primary lipoprotein lipase deficiency
4. Genetic absence of lipoprotein lipase activator } impaired lipoprotein lipase mediated triglyceride removal – very rare

SECONDARY – common

1. Obesity ⎫
2. Diabetes ⎪
3. Alcoholism ⎬ TG raised
4. Liver disease ⎪
5. Oestrogen therapy ⎪
6. Chronic renal failure ⎭
7. Hypothyroidism ⎫
8. Nephrotic syndrome ⎬ TG and CH raised
9. Renal transplantation ⎪
10. CAPD treatment ⎭

Causes of changes in total serum protein concentration

RAISED

1. Prolonged venous stasis before venepuncture – most common
2. Dehydration
3. Chronic infection – TB, parasites, SBE
4. Autoimmune disease – SLE, RA, PSS
5. Cirrhosis – albumin usually reduced
6. Paraproteinaemias
7. Sarcoid – (raised α_2 and γ)
8. Laboratory error

REDUCED

1. Artefactual – blood taken from a 'drip' arm
2. Excessive intravenous fluid
3. Reduced protein synthesis

   i. malnutrition
   ii. liver disease – albumen ↓
   iii. malabsorption
   iv. severe illness

4. Increased protein loss

   i. burns
   ii. nephrotic syndrome
   iii. protein-losing enteropathy
   iv. chronic peritoneal dialysis

Causes of osteoporosis

DEFINITION

A reduction in bone mass per unit volume with maintenance of normal mineral content. Appears to be related to increased bone resorption. There is no specific point of differentiation between normal and osteoporotic.

PRIMARY

1. Postmenopausal } as judged by the age when diagnosed.
2. Senile   } Concentrations of serum calcium, phospate
                     and alkaline phosphatase are *normal*

SECONDARY – much less frequent causes. Biochemical features variable

1. Corticosteroid treatment – irreversible in adults
2. Hyperparathyroidism
3. Hyperthyroidism – longstanding cases
4. Immobilization
5. Alcoholism
6. Hypogonadal states
7. Chronic renal failure – but often with osteitis fibrosa and osteomalacia
8. Bone metastases and multiple myeloma – usually focal lesion but generalized osteoporosis occurs

Causes of osteomalacia

DEFINITION

A reduction in mineral content of bone per unit mass of bone because of increased unmineralized matrix (osteoid). A deficiency of vitamin D in most cases. Rickets in childhood.

BIOCHEMICAL FEATURES

1. Serum alkaline phosphatase: almost always increased
2. Serum calcium: usually low or low normal
3. Serum phosphate

  i. either low or normal; tends to be inversely proportional to serum calcium concentration; secondary hyperparathyroidism tends to maintain the concentration of serum calcium which causes hypophosphataemia by the phosphaturic action of PTH
  ii. prominent hypophosphataemia occurs in Fanconi syndrome and hypophosphataemic rickets because of high renal phosphate clearance

DEFICIENT SUPPLY OF VITAMIN D

1. Elderly people eating restricted diet
2. Premature infants
3. Asian immigrants in Britain (inadequate exposure to sunlight)

IMPAIRED 25-HYDROXYLATION OF VITAMIN D $(25(OH)D_3)$

Chronic severe parenchymal liver disease

IMPAIRED Iα-HYDROXYLATION OF VITAMIN D $(1,25(OH)_2D_3)$

Chronic renal failure – GFR persistently <10 ml/min

IMPAIRED VITAMIN D ABSORPTION

Severe malabsorption states

OTHER CAUSES

1. Severe epileptics on high-dose anticonvulsants
2. Renal tubular acidosis and Fanconi syndrome – both rare
3. Familial hypophosphataemic rickets – rare

Paget's disease (osteitis deformans)

Unknown cause but perhaps an osteoclastic disorder. A disease of older age groups. Almost as common as osteoporosis. There is excessive and disorganized reabsorption and formation of one or many bones; never the entire skeleton. Has to be differentiated from osteomalacia and carcinoma of the prostate with osteosclerotic skeletal secondaries.

BIOCHEMICAL FEATURES

1. Serum alkaline phosphatase may be very high ($>300\,iu/\ell$, normal not more than 140) if many bones are involved by active disease. Rapidly increasing serum activity suggests possible development of an osteogenic sarcoma (but occurs in <1% of those with symptoms)
2. Serum calcium and phosphate concentrations normal
3. Serum acid phosphatase slightly increased (from osteoclasts)
4. Urinary hydroxyproline concentrations raised in proportion to serum alkaline phosphatase activity

Causes of hyperoxaluria

1. Increased ingestion or absorption of oxalate
   i. enteric hyperoxaluria
       (a) ileal by-pass surgery
       (b) ileo-colic fistulae
       (c) ileostomy
       (d) ileal resection
       the most common causes. In the presence of malabsorption, fat in the gut binds Ca^{2+} resulting in less Ca^{2+} to bind oxalate which is absorbed
   ii. excessive rhubarb

2. Ingestion of oxalate precursors
   i.   methoxyflurane
   ii. ethylene glycol – usually fatal
   iii. ascorbic acid
3. Increased endogenous production
   i. primary hyperoxaluria types I and II – very rare
   ii. pyridoxine deficiency

Drugs causing sodium and water retention

1. Steroids
   i.   all mineralocorticoids and corticosteriods
   ii. fludrocortisone – the most potent
   iii. anabolic steroids – occasionally
2. Oestrogens
   i. natural and synthetic oestrogens
   ii. stilboestrol – the most potent
3. Non-steroidal anti-inflammatory drugs – mild
4. Carbenoxolene and other liquorice-related compounds
5. Arteriolar vasodilators
   i.   minoxidil ⎱ very potent
   ii. diazoxide ⎰
   iii. nifedipine – quite potent
   iv. hydralazine – occasionally
6. Other hypotensive drugs
   i.   guanethidine ⎱ especially at start of therapy when a large
   ii. debrisoquine ⎰ fall in pressure may occur
   iii. methyldopa   ⎱ occasionally
   iv. β-blockers   ⎰
7. Sodium loading may occur when using
   i.   sodium bicarbonate
   ii. high dose sodium salts of penicillin or fusidic acid –
        especially in patients with chronic renal failure
   iii. sodium based X-ray contrast media

Useful blood tests in an alcoholic

1. Macrocytosis ⎱ without anaemia – occurs in >90%
2. Raised MCV ⎰
3. Raised γGT and AST
4. Reduced serum albumin   ⎱ established liver disease
5. Elevated alkaline phosphatase ⎰

Polydypsia and polyuria

>3ℓ urine daily; listed in frequency of occurrence

1. Diuretic treatment
2. Uncontrolled diabetes mellitus
3. Postobstructive diuresis
4. Chronic renal failure
5. Diuretic phase of acute renal failure
6. Prolonged lithium therapy
7. Hypercalcaemia or hypokalaemia
   (prolonged)

} all may be associated with varying degrees of renal impairment

8. Pituitary diabetes insipidus } infrequent; urine volume may
9. Compulsive water drinking } exceed 9ℓ daily

Diabetes insipidus

Cranial; pituitary; neurogenic (*see* page 172)

NEPHROGENIC

1. Familial – X-linked
2. Drug induced

   i.   lithium carbonate } used in the treatment
   ii. demeclocyclin HCl } of SIADH (*see* page 68)
   iii. amphotericin B

3. Metabolic

   i. hypokalaemia } occasionally if
   ii. hypercalcaemia } prolonged

Chapter 7

Renal diseases

Causes of unusually coloured urine

TABLE 7.1

Colour	Cause
Red	Haemoglobin, blood or myoglobinuria
	Rifampicin therapy
	Phenophthalein in alkaline urine
	Desferrioxamine
Orange	Concentrated
	Bile
Green/blue	Amitriptyline
	Methylene blue ingestion
Blue/black	Methaemoglobinuria
	Melanin
	Homogentisic acid–alkaptonuria
Cloudy	Urate
	Phosphate
	White blood cells
	Bacteria
Pale	Diuresis
	Chronic renal failure

Assessment of glomerular function

1. Plasma urea – inaccurate and may be misleading. Blood concentration altered by protein in diet, urine flow rate, catabolism in fever, digestion of blood in gut and occasionally liver failure
2. Plasma electrolytes – almost no relationship to GFR
3. Serum creatinine – a much more constant blood concentration is maintained than for urea
   Serum creatinine increased in:
   i. muscular men
   ii. transiently after a large meat meal

Blood concentration apparently increased by substances which interfere with:

i. the chemical analysis – ketones, glucose, hyperbilirubinaemia and rifampicin

ii. tubular secretion impaired – salicylates, cimetidine, trimethoprim

Blood concentration low in:

i. children, the elderly and patients with wasting diseases

ii. small women

4. Creatinine clearance is the ideal method of assessing GFR but urine collections are always suspect

5. For routine purposes clearance should be estimated from a formula, the best one being

$$\frac{88\ (145 - \text{age})}{\text{serum creatinine}} \times \frac{\text{weight (kg)}}{70} - 3$$

which expresses clearance in ml/minute/70 kg. For women the constant 88 has to be replaced by 75. The formula overestimates clearance when a subject weighs more than 80 kg

Causes of acute renal failure (ARF)

DEFINITION

Sudden (hours) reduction in urine flow such that the daily volume is less than 500 ml (<20 ml hourly). Urine osmolality is about 300–320 mmol/ℓ, urine Na is >60 mmol/ℓ and the urine/plasma osmolar (U/P) ratio is 1.3 or less.

There are four main groups of causes

1. Infections especially Gram negative bacteria – often coexists with hypotension

2. Low blood pressure – systolic <80 mmHg for some hours

3. Direct nephrotoxins

4. Acute obstruction to the flow of urine – this is not acute parenchymal failure but obstructive renal failure. Nevertheless obstruction must be excluded in all new patients with ARF

1. Infections
   i.   Gram negative septicaemia
   ii. infected burns
   iii. clostridial infections
   iv. *Legionella pneumophila*

2. Hypotension – loss of circulating volume
   i. severe burns – plasma loss
   ii. major gut haemorrhage

    iii. severe diarrhoea or vomiting
    iv. severe LVF – cardiogenic shock
    v. multiple fractures
    vi. ruptured aortic aneurysm
3. Nephrotoxins
    i.   gentamicin and other aminoglycosides
    ii. myoglobinuria – often associated with major trauma and infection
    iii. bilirubin – ARF occurs more readily after operations in jaundiced patients
    iv. paracetamol overdose
    v. paraquat and phenol
    vi. ethylene glycol – antifreeze
    vii. carbon tetrachloride
    viii. contrast media
4. Obstruction
    i.   pure acute obstruction causes anuria
    ii. intermittent obstruction may mimic the oliguria of ARF

ADVERSE PROGNOSTIC FEATURES OF ACUTE RENAL FAILURE

1. Presence of infection – especially septicaemias
2. Severe burns – >70 per cent body surface area
3. Rapidly rising urea >16 mmol/24 hour (>100 mg/100 ml per day)
4. Age >50 years
5. Oliguria >2 weeks
6. Other serious coexistent disease
7. Ventilation for >48 hours
8. By-pass surgery
9. Delay in starting active management

Early complications of acute renal failure

1. Plasma K^+ rising rapidly
2. Infections
3. Gut bleeds

Indications for dialysis in ARF

Clinical:
1. Poor clinical state, nausea, confusion
2. Fluid overload, pulmonary oedema
3. To accommodate crystalloid, colloid or TPN solutions
Biochemical:
1. Plasma K^+ >7.5 mmol/ℓ and rising
2. Plasma urea >35 mmol/ℓ (200 mg/100 ml)
3. Plasma bicarbonate <12 mmol/ℓ or arterial pH <7.15

4. Plasma urea rising >16 mmol/ℓ per day (100 mg/100 ml). 'Hypercatabolic' acute renal failure

Often more than one indication is present at the same time. Hyperkalaemia is the usual indication for emergency dialysis.

Major causes of chronic renal failure (CRF)

These conditions do not all necessarily lead to death from renal failure.

1. Chronic glomerulonephritis –
   including collagen diseases } the major causes
2. Diabetes mellitus
3. Chronic obstructive uropathy*
4. Hypertension – also often complicates other causes of CRF
5. Polycystic renal disease – accounts for about 10 per cent of a chronic dialysis population
6. Chronic pyelonephritis and other interstitial nephritides
7. Renal tuberculosis*
8. Miscellaneous
   i.   amyloid
   ii. analgesic nephropathy*
   iii. vitamin D (or analogues) excess*
   iv. urate nephropathy*
   v.   sarcoid*
   vi. hyperparathyroidism*

Presenting features of polycystic renal disease

1. Abdominal mass
2. Hypertension
3. Haematuria   } both may also be associated with
4. Urinary tract infection } renal pain
5. Chronic renal failure

Causes of obstruction to the urinary tract

Obstruction often develops slowly; the volume of urine may not, at first, be altered. Acute anuria is quite infrequent.

1. Enlarged prostate – the most common
2. Carcinoma of the bladder obstructing ureteric orifices
3. Renal calculi in both kidneys, both ure-   } explains about
   ters, in one kidney and the ureter of the   } 90 per cent
   other side or in an anatomically or func-   } of cases
   tionally single kidney

* potentially treatable

4. Following pelvic surgery with cutting or tying off of both ureters
5. Retroperitoneal fibrosis
6. Sudden precipitation of urate or sulphonamide crystals in both pelves or ureters, or both
7. Sloughed papillae obstructing ureters ⎫
8. Oedema of ureters following retrograde pyelography ⎬ rare

Causes of acute anuria

No urine formed.

1. Mechanical – causes 2–8 above ⎫
2. Renal parenchymal
   i.   acute glomerulonephritis
   ii. acute interstitial nephritis ⎬ rare
3. Renal vascular
   i.   thrombosis of renal veins or arteries
   ii. severe trauma to both kidneys ⎭

Clinical features of CRF

These develop only when the plasma urea is persistently above 50 mmol/ℓ (300 mg/100 ml)

1. Gastrointestinal*
   i.   nausea ⎫
   ii. vomiting ⎬ very common, controllable by diet at first
   iii. anorexia
2. Cardiovascular
   i.   hypertension – very common*
   ii. atheroma
   iii. pericarditis – pre-terminal*
   iv. pericardial effusion – transudate or bloody*
3. Respiratory system*
   i.   acidotic respiration – pre-terminal
   ii. tachypnoea
        (a) secondary to anaemia
        (b) if fluid overloaded
4. Anaemia – normal indices; major cause of ill health in CRF
5. Skin
   i.   muddy yellow-brown
   ii. pale – anaemia
   iii. scratch marks
   iv. easily bronzed by sun

* controllable by dialysis

6. Nervous system*
   i. headaches and impaired concentration
   ii. peripheral neuropathy
   iii. fits
   iv. myopathy

7. Bones and calcium metabolism†
   i. secondary hyperparathyroidism – fingers, rugger-jersey spine
   ii. osteomalacia
   iii. osteoporosis
   iv. soft tissue calcification

Laboratory variables at different degrees of CRF

Note that concentrations of many variables begin to change to a major degree only as the GFR falls to <20 ml/min.

TABLE 7.2

Variables	Normal (N)	Mild	Moderate	Advanced	Terminal
GFR ml/min	125–80	80–40	40–20	20–10	<3
Hb g/dl(g/100 ml)	18–12	N	12–8	8–6	<6
Indices	N	N	N	N	N
WBC × 10^9/ℓ/(/mm³)	N	N	N	N	N
Urea mmol/ℓ	3.3–6.6	N	8–15.0	15–40	50–100
(mg/100 ml)	20–40		50–90	90–250	300–600
Creatinine					
μmol/ℓ	50–130	N	140–250	250–400	1000–2000
(mg/100 ml)	0.6–1.5		1.6–2.8	2.8–4.5	11.3–22.6
Na mmol/ℓ(mEq/ℓ)	135–146	N	N	N	125–135
K mmol/ℓ (mEq/ℓ)	3.5–5.5	N	N	N	>7.0
Bicarbonate					
mmol/ℓ (mEq/ℓ)	22–28	N	20–15	15–10	<10
Calcium mmol/ℓ	2.25–2.6	N	N	2.0–2.2	<1.9
(mg/100 ml)	9–10.5			8.0–8.8	<7.6
Phosphate mmol/ℓ	0.7–1.4	N	1.4–2.0	2.0–4.0	>4.5
(mg/100 ml)	2.2–4.3		4.3–6.2	6.2–12.4	>14.0
Urate mmol/ℓ	0.2–0.39	N	N	0.5–0.8	>1.2
(mg/100 ml)	3.5–6.5			8.5–13.5	>20.0
Arterial pH	7.36–7.42	N	N	7.3–7.2	<7.1
nmol/ℓ	36–43			50–60	>80

* controllable by dialysis
† controllable by metabolic means or surgery

Hypokalaemia with renal failure

Patients with renal failure tend to have normal or raised plasma K^+ concentrations. Some, a few, do not

1. Excessive diuretic usage
2. Secondary hyperaldosteronism
3. K^+ loss from gut
4. Renal tubular acidosis
5. Correction of acidosis without K^+ replacement

Causes of proteinuria

Virtually all diseases of the kidney and the urinary tract cause an increase above the normal protein excretion of 100–200 mg/day.

Four general groups are definable

1. Tubular proteinuria – about 1 g/day and in particular containing an increased quantity of β_2 microglobulin
2. Proteinuria of 1–2 g daily. Found in non-glomerular parenchymal diseases such as acute and chronic infections
3. Proteinuria of >4 g daily – glomerular lesions in particular glomerulonephritis
4. Bence-Jones proteinuria – free light chains of immunoglobulins found in
   i.   myeloma
   ii. amyloid
   iii. Waldenström's macroglobulinaemia ⎫
   iv. lymphoma   ⎬ rare
   v.   chronic lymphatic leukaemia   ⎭

Causes of haematuria

Multiple possible causes; the main ones are

1. Cancer of
   i.   bladder   ⎫ 'painless   ⎫ the majority
   ii. kidney   ⎬ haematuria'   ⎬ of patients
   iii. pelvis or ureters ⎭ |
2. Pelvic and ureteric stones   ⎭
3. Acute pyelonephritis
4. Glomerulonephritides
5. Trauma to renal tract
6. Enlarged prostate
7. Polycystic renal disease
8. SBE
9. Factitious
10. Infarction
11. Sickle-cell disease

Classification of the glomerulonephritides

1. Minimal change – major cause of nephrotic syndrome in children ⎫
2. Membranous – chronic proteinuria in adults ⎬ specific diseases
3. Focal segmental – proteinuria and haematuria ⎭
4. Proliferative

   i. acute exudative – acute nephritis
   ii. mesangial
   iii. mesangiocapillary – often with complement abnormalities
   iv. focal – the morphological finding in Henoch–Schönlein nephritis, SLE and polyarteritis nodosa
   v. extracapillary – >70 per cent crescents – rare, with rapid loss of function
   vi. advanced sclerosing and unclassifiable – found in patients with advanced renal failure

Clinical syndromes of glomerulonephritis

1. Persistent proteinuria
2. Nephrotic syndrome
3. Recurrent haematuria
4. Acute nephritic syndrome
5. Chronic renal failure

while these syndromes are presented as separate entities, often overlapping features are present. No specific glomerular morphology necessarily characterizes any particular syndrome

Antigens of glomerular nephritis

The casual antigens in the majority of nephritides have not been found.

1. Infectious agents

   i. streptococci
   ii. staphylococci
   iii. quartan malaria
   iv. *Treponema pallidum*
   v. *M. leprae*
   vi. schistosomiasis
   vii. hepatitis B
   viii. cytomegalovirus (CMV)

2. Drugs

   i. penicillamine
   ii. gold
   iii. probenicid – and many others

3. Miscellaneous
   i. DNA
   ii. tumour antigens
   iii. glomerular basement membrane

Causes of nephrotic syndrome

DEFINITION

Pitting oedema, hypoalbuminaemia, proteinuria >4 g/day

1. Glomerulonephritides – 80–90 per cent of all cases (including collagen vascular diseases)
2. Metabolic diseases
   i. diabetes mellitus ⎱ account for 5–10 per cent of adult
   ii. amyloid ⎰ nephrotics
3. Drugs
   i. gold ⎱ best examples, but infrequently occur
   ii. penicillamine ⎰
   iii. captopril
   iv. troxidone
   v. street heroin
4. Infections
   i. hepatitis B
   ii. malaria
   iii. SBE
5. Neoplasia
   i. carcinoma
   ii. lymphoma
6. Renal vein thrombosis – usually secondary to a pre-existing glomerular lesion

Common histological patterns in nephrotics

TABLE 7.3

Histology	Likely age of patient (years)
Minimal change	1–10
Mesangiocapillary	10–20
Focal	15–30
Membranous	25–50

Frequency of presentations and likely outcomes of some nephritides
TABLE 7.4

	Persistent proteinuria	Nephrotic syndrome	Recurrent haematuria	Acute nephritis	Chronic renal failure
Minimal change		+++			
IgA/C3 (Berger's)			+++		±
Acute exudative		+		+++	
Mesangiocapillary	+	++		+	++
Membranous	+++	++			++
Focal		+	+	+	+
Extracapillary crescents	++		++		+++
Lupus nephritis	++	++			++

Key to symbols: +++ = invariable; ++ = very frequent; + = often; ± = infrequent

Indications for a renal biopsy

1. Nephrotic syndrome in all patients over the age of 12 years with the possible exception of diabetics
2. Persistent proteinuria of >1 g daily; assuming smooth renal outlines on IVU
3. Recurrent haematuria particularly in adults – after a neoplasm has been excluded
4. Systemic diseases such as lupus and polyarteritis nodosa with renal involvement – for diagnostic and prognostic purposes
5. Chronic renal failure – providing the GFR is >10 ml/min
6. Impairment of transplant kidney function
7. Unexplained acute renal failure
8. Serial biopsy to study natural history or response to treatment

Contra-indications to a renal biopsy

1. Uncontrolled hypertension
2. Single functioning kidney – except in the case of a graft kidney
3. Coagulation defect
4. Obstructive uropathy
5. Lack of patient cooperation

Causes of renal vein thrombosis

Quite an unusual condition, most commonly is secondary to membranous nephropathy

1. Complication of a nephrotic state   } the two
2. Renal amyloid – intrarenal thrombosis   } most common

3. Growth of a hypernephroma into the renal vein
4. Complicating severe dehydration in infants
5. Trauma to renal vein

    i. indwelling cannulae
    ii. external pressure due to enlarged nodes

Tubulointerstitial nephritis (interstitial nephritis)

A heterogeneous group of conditions chiefly involving the renal interstitium and tubules.
Glomeruli are not primarily involved and proteinuria is <2 g/day.

ACUTE

1. Acute bacterial pyelonephritis – easily the most common
2. Acute drug hypersensitivity reaction

    i.   methicillin
    ii. rifampicin
    iii. phenindione
    iv. thiazides

3. Legionnaires' disease
4. Leukaemic infiltration
5. Idiopathic

CHRONIC

1. Chronic pyelonephritis   } the most common
2. Vesico-ureteric reflux
3. Analgesic nephropathy
4. Urate nephropathy
5. Transplant rejection
6. Tubulo-interstitial injury associated with glomerulonephritis
7. Sarcoid and leprosy
8. Radiation nephritis
9. Idiopathic

Renal tubular disorders

Many are rare.

IMPAIRED REABSORPTION

1. Water

    i. nephrogenic diabetes insipidus
    ii. compulsive water drinking – acquired deficiency

2. Glucose – renal glycosuria   } the three most common
3. Calcium – idiopathic hypercalciuria
4. Amino acids – cystinuria

5. Sodium and potassium – distal tubular damage due to
   i. renal stones
   ii. papillary necrosis
6. Phosphate, glucose, potassium and amino acids
   i. some cases of myeloma damaged kidneys
   ii. adult Fanconi syndrome
   iii. heavy metal (Hg, Pb) poisoning

INABILITY TO ACIDIFY

1. Renal tubular acidosis
2. Distal tubular damage due to
   i. lithium carbonate – not uncommon
   ii. hypokalaemia ⎫
   iii. hypercalcaemia ⎬ prolonged
   iv. stones, papillary necrosis, hydronephrosis

Renal associations of polycythaemia

1. Polycystic disease – often
2. Transplanted kidneys ⎫
3. Hypernephroma ⎬ occasionally
4. Hydronephrosis ⎭

Classification of renal cysts

1. Single, or 2 to 3 – quite common in adults, often found by chance
2. Multiple
   i. polycystic renal disease – adult (quite common) and infantile varieties (fatal)
   ii. cystic dysplasia ⎫
   iii. small cysts in various hereditary disorders ⎬ rare

Causes of enlarged kidneys

Normal length is 11–14 cm in an adult.

UNILATERAL

1. Renal cyst or cysts
2. Compensatory hypertrophy
3. Unilateral duplex kidney
4. Neoplasm (Wilms' tumour, hypernephroma)
5. Pyonephrosis

BILATERAL

1. Early insulin-dependent diabetes
2. Bilateral hydronephrosis
3. Acute parenchymal disease
    i.   nephrotic syndrome
    ii. acute renal failure
    iii. acute interstitial nephritides
    iv. acute pyelonephritis
4. Polycystic renal disease
5. Bilateral duplex collecting systems
6. Acromegaly – rare

Causes of small kidneys

UNILATERAL

1. Reflux uropathy
2. Postobstructive atrophy
3. Postinfarction or venous thrombosis
4. Congenital hypoplasia
5. Tuberculosis
6. Renal artery stenosis

BILATERAL – chronic renal failure of any cause

Causes of sterile pyuria

1. Renal tuberculosis – not uncommon
2. Persistent inflammation as with renal stones
3. Analgesic nephropathy – becoming more common
4. Non-specific inflammation of bladder

Causes of papillary necrosis

Not common

1. Obstructive uropathy – particularly if infected
2. Renal tuberculosis
3. Acute pyelonephritis – especially in diabetics
4. Sickle cell disease and other haemoglobinopathies
5. Analgesic nephropathy
6. Dysproteinaemias

Factors associated with urinary infections

1. Sexual intercourse in females
2. Pregnancy – progesterone dilatation of collecting tract
3. Obstruction to urine flow
4. Catheterization or instrumentation of bladder
5. Diabetes mellitus
6. Renal stones
7. Papillary necrosis
8. Structural abnormalities of the urinary tract – leading to obstruction, reflux or both

Nephrocalcinosis and renal calcification

1. All causes of hypercalciuria if sufficiently prolonged – (*see* page 69)
2. Renal tuberculosis
3. Renal tubular acidosis
4. Cortical necrosis – old
5. Calcification in a cyst, haematoma or renal carcinoma
6. Medullary sponge kidney
7. Oxalosis

} rare

DEFINITIONS

Bacteriuria
Bacteria in urine other than urethral flora. A laboratory finding which may or may not be accompanied by symptoms.

Covert bacteriuria
Bacteriuria without symptoms.

Urinary tract infection
Bacteria recovered from the urine in significant numbers ($>100\,000\,mm^3$) with renal tract signs or symptoms or both. No specific site of infection is implied.

Composition of renal stones

Crystals (97.5 per cent) deposited upon a matrix (2.5 per cent). Matrix is composed of protein, sugars, glucosamine, carbon dioxide and water.

TABLE 7.5

Crystal components	Frequency (%)	Radio-opacity
Calcium oxalate ± phosphate	65–70	Opaque
Calcium phosphate – apatite	15	Opaque
Magnesium–ammonium–phosphate – MAP; struvite (infection associated)	10–15	Opaque
Uric acid	5	Not opaque
Cystine	2	Mildly opaque
Xanthine	<0.01	Radiolucent

Investigation of a renal stone

1. Blood
   i. fasting, non-stasis Ca^{2+}, phosphate and albumin $\times$ 2
   ii. uric acid
   iii. PTH – selected cases only

2. Urine
   i. microscopy and culture – an excess of non-glomerular erythrocytes are found with stones and pyuria
   ii. overnight fasting pH
   iii. two consecutive 24-hour urine saves for Ca^{2+} and uric acid
   iv. creatinine clearance
   v. cystine screen
   vi. oxalate excretion – children chiefly

3. X-rays
   i. plain abdominal film
   ii. IVU
   iii. retrograde pyelography in some
   iv. CT scan – occasionally

Drugs and the kidney

ACUTE LESIONS

1. Acute tubular necrosis – direct toxic effect

   i. aminoglycosides – quite common
   ii. solvents – carbon tetrachloride, glycols
   iii. cisplatin
   iv. heavy metals – mercury, bismuth   } infrequent
   v. snake venom
   vi. some mushroom toxins

2. Acute interstitial nephritis
    i.   sulphonamides
    ii. ampicillin
    iii. rifampicillin
    iv. thiazides
3. Drug-induced lupus-like state – *see* page 270
    i.   hydralazine – slow acetylators
    ii. isoniazid
    iii. procainamide
    iv. oral contraceptives
4. Acute obstruction – intra-renal
    i.   cytotoxics leading to urate precipitation in distal tubular lumena when patients are not protected by allopurinol
    ii. X-ray contrast and dehydration leading to precipitation of Bence-Jones protein
    iii. sulphonamide crystalluria – infrequent

LESIONS LEADING TO IMPAIRED FUNCTION

1. Immune complex glomerulonephritis
    i.   gold, penicillamine $\Big\}$ nephrotic state
    ii. troxidone, tolbutamide
2. Analgesic nephropathy – infrequent; NSAIDs are now the principal drugs involved
3. Disturbance of protein metabolism
    i.   tetracycline in patients with chronic renal failure impairs amino acid incorporation into protein. The amino acids are deaminated leading to an increase in the plasma urea concentration
    ii. Steroids also cause divergence in the urea: creatinine in ratio
4. Retroperitoneal fibrosis
    i.   methysergide – rarely used in patients with migraine
    ii. practolol – now withdrawn   NB oculomucocutaneous syndrome
5. Hypercalcaemia – secondary to excess vitamin D (may persist for months after stopping the drug) or analogues of vitamin D (much shorter duration of hypercalcaemia – few weeks after withdrawal)
6. Hyperuricaemia – secondary to cytotoxic therapy of reticuloses

DRUGS CAUSING HYPOKALAEMIA

1. Diuretics
2. Prolonged steroid therapy – Na^+ retention with K^+ loss
3. Carbenoxolone
4. Laxative abuse
5. Excessive ingestion of liquorice

ADH AND THE KIDNEY

Loss of concentrating ability
  i. lithium salts
  ii. NSAIDs
  iii. amphotericin B
  iv. hypercalcaemia ⎫ prolonged
  v. hypokalaemia   ⎭
  vi. methoxyflurane

HYPO- AND HYPERVOLAEMIA AND RENAL IMPAIRMENT

1. Sodium and water depletion
  i. secondary to drugs causing prolonged vomiting or diarrhoea
  ii. excessive use of i.v. loop diuretics
2. Hypernatraemia and hypertension
  i. carbenicillin ⎫ due to high sodium content
  ii. fusidic acid ⎭

DRUG COMBINATIONS

1. Cephaloridine and frusemide ⎫ tubular necrosis
2. Gentamicin and frusemide   ⎭
3. Probenicid and cytotoxics – urate sludge
4. Fixed diuretic–potassium sparing combinations
  i. amiloride   ⎫ with thiazides may lead to hyperkalaemia
  ii. triamterine ⎬ if given to patients with impaired renal
  iii. sprinolactone ⎭ function

Renal disease, haemolytic anaemia and thrombocytopenia

1. SLE
2. Pre-eclampsia and obstetric accidents
3. Oral contraceptives

4. Haemolytic uraemic syndrome ⎤
5. Malignant hypertension   ⎥
6. Cardiac prostheses   ⎬ uncommon
7. Disseminated carcinoma   ⎥
8. Mismatched blood transfusion   ⎦

Causes of a false positive sulfosalicylic acid test for urine protein

1. X-ray contrast media
2. Penicillins
3. Co-trimoxazole metabolites
4. Tolbutamide metabolites
5. Para-aminosalicylic acid
6. Metabolites of tolmetin sodium – a NSAID

Causes of urinary incontinence

Most common in elderly people

1. Diuresis – loop diuretics, glycosuria
2. Neurological – UMN lesions, autonomic denervation as in diabetics
3. Dementia
4. Sedatives and antidepressants – particularly in the elderly
5. Acute confusional states seen in acute infections
6. Urinary tract infections or interstitial cystitis
7. Attention seeking

ADDITIONAL FEATURES IN WOMEN

1. Prolapse
    i.   uterus   ⎤
    ii. cystocele   ⎬ stress incontinence due to
    iii. urethrocele   ⎦ sphincteric weakness
2. Malignant fistulae
    i.   vesico-vaginal
    ii. uretero-vaginal
3. Ectopic ureter in young girls (rare)

ADDITIONAL FEATURES IN MEN

1. Prostate
    i.   hypertrophy with retention and overflow
    ii. post-prostatectomy
2. Urethral stricture

Renal transplantation
TABLE 7.6

Advantages	Disadvantages
1. Restoration to a virtually normal life 2. No fluid restriction 3. No dialysis 4. Ability to travel freely 5. Restoration of fertility 6. Able to work full-time 7. Cheaper for the DHSS	1. Complications of steroids – *see* page 305 2. Possibility of opportunistic infections 3. Increased chance of lymphomas – 30 per cent intracerebral 4. Anxiety regarding function of graft 5. Suitable organs in short supply

Uses of peritoneal dialysis

1. Chronic renal failure – Continuous Ambulatory Peritoneal Dialysis (CAPD)
2. Acute renal failure
3. Emergency control of hyperkalaemia
4. Diuretic resistent acute pulmonary oedema
5. Correction of severe hyponatraemia or hypercalcaemia – occasionally
6. Removal of water soluble poisons

    i.   salicylates
    ii. long acting barbiturates   } very occasionally
    iii. ethanol, methanol

Advantages and disadvantages of CAPD
TABLE 7.7

Advantages	Disadvantages
1. Training and establishing at home takes 2–3 weeks 2. No machinery or modification of the home needed 3. No help required 4. Fluid and food restriction less severe than for haemodialysis 5. Haemoglobin rises to about 10 g/dl in the first 3 months of therapy 6. Treatment of choice for diabetics 7. Improved growth rates in children compared with haemodialysis 8. Usually good phosphate control and perhaps less osteodystrophy	1. Bacterial peritonitis a major complication 2. Repetitive technique proves very boring for some patients 3. May be quite time consuming (four exchanges daily) 4. Persistent hypertriglyceridaemia results 5. Weight gain may occur as a consequence of hypertonic dialysate 6. Loss of serum protein across peritoneal membrane 7. Abdominal catheter may prove sexually inhibiting 8. Increased incidence of inguinal hernias and perhaps gastro-oseophageal reflux

Chapter 8

Haematology

Substances needed for erythropoiesis

1. Hormones – erythropoietin, thyroxine, androgens
2. Vitamins – B_{12}, B_6, folate, C, thiamine, riboflavin, pantothenic acid
3. Metals – Fe, Mn, Co.

Normal human haemoglobins

TABLE 8.1

Haemoglobin	Chain structure	Percentage of normal adult haemoglobin	Percentage of haemoglobin at birth
A	$\alpha2$ $\beta2$	97.0	10–50
A_2	$\alpha2$ $\delta2$	2.5	Trace
F	$\alpha2$ $\gamma2$	0.5	50–90

Anaemia

If the haemoglobin is less than the figures quoted below, an anaemia is present

Adult male   15.5
Adult female   12.5
3 months to puberty   12.0 } g/dl (g/100 ml) of whole blood
Neonates   19.0

Note

1. Reduction in plasma volume, as in dehydration, may mask an anaemia

2. An expanded circulating volume (such as occurs following over infusion of fluids) will cause an anaemia despite a normal total circulating red cell and haemoglobin mass
3. Following acute major blood loss (such as variceal bleeding), there is no apparent anaemia because the total blood volume is reduced. When the circulating volume is repleted the anaemia becomes apparent. *See Table 8.2,* below

Relationship between red cell and plasma volumes

TABLE 8.2

Red cell volume (25–30 ml/kg)	Plasma volume (45 ml/kg)	Cause		Effect
Normal	High	i.	Pregnancy (third trimester)	Relative anaemia
		ii.	Congestive heart failure	
		iii.	Cirrhosis	
		iv.	Fluid overload	
Normal	Low	i.	Peripheral circulatory failure	Relative polycythaemia
		ii.	Dehydration	
		iii.	High altitude	
		iv.	Excess diuretic therapy	
Low	Normal	Anaemia		Normal for slowly developing anaemia
Low	High	Anaemia		Anaemia less severe than indicated by blood count
Low	Low	Anaemia (severe)		Blood count under estimating degree of anaemia
High	High	Polycythaemia		Defect more severe than apparent
Normal	Normal or low	i.	Polycythaemia vera	Correct reflection of clinical condition
		ii.	Secondary polycythaemia	

Classification of anaemias

BLOOD LOSS

1. Acute
2. Chronic

the most common causes world wide; they are due to reduced red cell production, an increased rate of destruction or loss of erythrocytes from the circulation

IMPAIRED RED CELL FORMATION

1. Acquired deficiencies of haematinics
   i.   iron – very common world wide
   ii. vitamin B_{12} or folic acid – megaloblastic, *see* page 103
2. Anaemias unrelated to genetic errors or haematinic deficiency
   i.   secondary to
        (a) metastatic malignant disease – not necessarily with
            marrow replacement
        (b) inflammatory disorders – RA, SLE, Crohn's disease
        (c) chronic infection – many causes
        (d) chronic renal or liver failure
   ii. endocrine diseases
        (a) myxoedema – common
        (b) hypopituitarism – rare
   iii. drug-induced
        (a) dose related cytotoxic therapy – common
        (b) idiosyncratic
   iv. infiltration of bone marrow
        (a) metastatic carcinoma – quite common
        (b) acute and chronic leukaemias
        (c) multiple myeloma
        (d) malignant lymphoma
        (e) myelofibrosis
   v.   aplastic anaemia – primary or secondary
   vi. refractory sideroblastic anaemia – rare

HAEMOLYTIC ANAEMIA

1. Acquired } *see* page 105
2. Inherited }

Classification of anaemias by red cell indices

1. Microcytic, hypochromic
   i.   iron deficiency } MCV   <80 fl (μm^3)
   ii. thalassaemia   } MCH   <27 pg ($\mu\mu g$)
   iii. sideroblastic   } MCHC <32 g/dl (g/100 ml)
2. Normocytic, normochromic
   i.   after acute blood loss
   ii. many chronic disorders – Hb   MCV 80–95 fl
        usually not <9 g/dl   MCH 27–32 pg
   iii. many haemolytic anaemias
3. Macrocytic – megaloblastic anaemias; MCV >100 fl

Causes of iron deficiency

1. Blood loss

   i. uterine – heavy or prolonged periods
   ii. gut
       (a) ulcers of stomach, duodenum or hiatus hernia
       (b) carcinoma of colon, rectum or stomach
       (c) inflammatory bowel disease – *see* page 145
       (d) gastric varices
       (e) infestations such as hookworms

2. Increased demand

   i. pregnancy or menstruation
   ii. growth

3. Poor diet – usually a contributory factor, not a sole cause
4. Malabsorption – majority of causes of malabsorption – *see* page 142

Sideroblastic anaemia

A refractory hypochromic anaemia. Dimorphic blood picture. Normal or raised serum iron. The marrow shows increased iron stores and many pathological ring sideroblasts – iron granules around the nucleus; uncommon.

1. Idiopathic – the most common
2. Secondary to

   i. (a) isoniazid – vitamin B_6 antagonist
       (b) alcohol
   ii. haematological
       (a) systemic
       (b) chronic inflammation
       (c) myelosclerosis

3. Hereditary – occurs in males transmitted by females, very rare

Failure of a hypochromic anaemia to respond to oral iron

1. Continued blood loss
2. Incorrect diagnosis – thalassaemia or sideroblastic anaemia
3. Mixed deficiency anaemia – B_{12} or folate deficient in addition
4. Failure to take tablets

Laboratory features of a hypochromic anaemia

TABLE 8.3

Laboratory variable	Iron deficiency	Chronic inflammation or malignancy	α or β thalassaemia trait	Sideroblastic anaemia
MCV	All ↓ according to degree of anaemia	Low normal or mild reduction	All ↓ or very reduced to degree of anaemia	MCV ↑ in acquired varieties
MCH				
MCHC				
Serum Fe	↓	↓	Normal	↑
TIBC	↑	↓	Normal	Normal
Serum ferritin	↓	Normal	Normal	↑
Bone marrow iron	↓ or nil	Normal	Normal	↑
Erythroblast	Absent	Absent	Normal	Ring sideroblasts
Haemoglobin electrophoresis	Normal	Normal	Abnormal	Normal

Causes of megaloblastic anaemia

Normochromic

  i. MCV 100–110 fl suggests liver disease, alcohol abuse, hypothyroidism or myeloma
 ii. MCV >110 fl suggests deficiency of B_{12} or folate

VITAMIN B_{12} DEFICIENCY

1. Inadequate diet – chiefly vegans (Hindu Indians)
2. Malabsorption
    i. gastric
        (a) pernicious anaemia – the most common cause in Western Europe
        (b) partial or total gastrectomy – takes 2–4 years to develop – B_{12} deficiency
        (c) congenital lack of intrinsic factor – rare
   ii. gut
        (a) B_{12} malabsorption:
            Crohn's disease
            ileal resection
            chronic tropical sprue
        (b) B_{12} utilization by bacteria or parasites:
            blind loop syndrome, jejunal diverticula, anatomical blind loops
            fish tape worm – in Finland and parts of the Far East

FOLATE DEFICIENCY

1. Nutritional – predisposing features
    i.   poverty
    ii. old age
    iii. alcoholism
2. Malabsorption – not common
    i.   gluten enteropathy – most common cause
    ii. tropical sprue
    iii. dermatitis herpetiformis
    iv. gastrectomy ⎫
    v.. extensive jejunal resection ⎬ may contribute in some patients
    vi.. Crohn's disease ⎭
3. Excessive requirements
    i.   physiological
         (a) pregnancy and lactation – requirements increase by a factor of 3 to 4
         (b) prematurity
    ii. pathological
         (a) haematological disease:
             haemolytic anaemias
             myelosclerosis
         (b) malignancy:
             carcinoma
             myeloma
             lymphoma
         (c) inflammatory diseases:
             rheumatoid arthritis
             psoriasis and other skin shedding conditions
             malaria
4. Drug causes
    i.   anticonvulsants and barbiturates
    ii. anti-folate drugs such as methotrexate, trimethoprim
    iii. sulphasalazine ⎫ impairs absorption
         cholestyramine ⎭
5. Mixed
    i.   alcoholism
    ii. oral contraceptives – never a main cause
    iii. liver disease

Indications for serum B_{12} assay

1. Megaloblastic anaemia
2. Macrocytic anaemia
3. Post-gastrectomy anaemia with hypersegmented polymorphs

4. Peripheral neuropathy
5. Dementia
6. Optic atrophy
7. Sub-acute combined degeneration of the cord

Causes of macrocytosis

MCV >100 fl

1. Vitamin B_{12} deficiency ⎫
2. Folate deficiency   ⎬ megaloblastic marrow
3. Blood regeneration – reticulocytes are larger ⎱
   than mature red cells
4. Alcoholism
5. Liver disease
6. Myeloma
7. Cytotoxic drug therapy   normoblastic
8. Leuco-erythroblastic anaemia   marrow
9. Myxoedema
10. Haemolysis – reticulocytes
11. Aplastic anaemia and red-cell aplasia
12. Idiopathic acquired sideroblastic anaemia

Causes of microcytosis

MCV <80 fl

1. Iron deficiency
2. Anaemia of chronic disorders
3. Thyrotoxicosis
4. α- or β-thalassaemia trait
5. Hereditary spherocytosis
6. Sideroblastic anaemia

Haemolytic anaemias

Anaemia only develops if red cell survival time is <15 days because a healthy marrow can compensate for increased loss of erythrocytes by an increase in production provided that there is an adequate supply of haematinics.

1. Acquired
   i.   infections – Gram-negative septicaemia (common), malaria, clostridial
   ii. disseminated intravascular coagulation – microangiopathic haemolytic anaemia (*see* page 121)
   iii. immune
        (a) autoimmune

    (b) drug-induced
    (c) haemolytic disease of the new born
    (d) haemolytic transfusion reactions
  iv. red cell fragmentation – mechanical damage; uncommon
   v. hypersplenism ⎫
  vi. haemolytic uraemic syndrome ⎬ rare
2. Inherited
   i. membrane defect ⎫
    (a) hereditary spherocytosis
    (b) hereditary elliptocytosis
   ii. metabolic defect ⎬ infrequent
    (a) glucose-6-phosphate dehydrogenase
      (G6PD) deficiency
    (b) pyruvate kinase (PK) deficiency ⎭
  iii. haemoglobin defect
    (a) abnormal – HbS, (the most common); Hb C, D or E
    (b) defective synthesis – thalassaemias

Laboratory features of haemolytic anaemias

BIOCHEMICAL

1. Serum unconjugated bilirubin ⎫
2. Urine urobilinogen
3. Faecal stercobilinogen ⎬ raised
4. Serum methaemalbumin ⎭
5. Haemosiderinuria
6. Serum haptoglobulins – absent; combines with free haemoglobin

HAEMATOLOGICAL

1. Reticulocytosis
2. Bone marrow erythroid hyperplasia
3. Red cell morphology – blood film
   i. spherocytes – immune haemolytic anaemia, hereditary
    spherocytosis, burns
   ii. target cells – thalassaemia, Hb C disease; obstructive
    jaundice
  iii. sickle cells – Hb S, S-C disease and in sickle-thalassaemia
   iv. Burr cells – chronic renal failure
   v. elliptocytes – hereditary elliptocytosis
   vi. fragments – microangiopathic haemolytic anaemia; DIC,
    accelerated hypertension, mechanical haemolysis
  vii. auto-agglutination – mycoplasmal infections

4. Coombs' test – detects antibody on red cells
5. Osmotic fragility
6. ^{51}Cr labelling of patient's cells

Intravascular haemolysis

The direct destruction of red cells in the circulation

CAUSES

1. Malaria – black water fever
2. ABO incompatible transfusion
3. G6PD deficiency
4. Paroxysmal nocturnal haemoglobinuria
5. Mechanical damage – March haemoglobinaemia, valve replacements except homografts, aortic >mitral, patch repair of a VSD, severe AS + AR

SPECIFIC LABORATORY FEATURES

1. Haemoglobulinaemia
2. Methaemoglobulinaemia – Schumm's test
3. Haemoglobulinuria
4. Haemosiderinuria
5. Fall or absence of serum haptoglobulin

Auto-immune haemolytic anaemias (AIHA)

WARM TYPES (37°C)

1. Idiopathic – diagnosis by exclusion
2. Secondary, circa 50 per cent, to
   i.   SLE
   ii. CLL and lymphomas
   iii. methyldopa

LABORATORY FEATURES

1. Direct Coombs' test positive with IgG, IgG and C3 or IgA on red cells
2. Best detected at 37°C

COLD TYPES (4°C)

1. Idiopathic – diagnosis by exclusion
2. Secondary to
   i.   infectious mononucleosis

    ii. mycoplasmal pneumonia
    iii. lymphomas
3. Paroxysmal cold haemoglobinuria – rare

LABORATORY FEATURES

1. Red cells agglutinate in the cold due to haemagglutinins which are IgM autoantibodies
2. Coombs' positive only with C3
3. Specific serum IgM against red cell antigen 'I' (*Mycoplasma pneumoniae*) or 'i' (EB infection)
4. Best detected at 4°C

Drug-induced Coombs' positive haemolysis

1. Lupus-like syndrome
    i.   hydralazine – in slow acetylators
    ii. procainamide
2. Antigen–antibody complex on RBC
    i.   phenacetin
    ii. chlorpromide
    iii. quinidine bisulphate
3. Attachment to RBC membrane
    i.   penicillin if $>20 \times 10^6$ units i.v. daily
    ii. cephalothin
4. Unexplained – methyldopa

Haemoglobinopathies

A hereditary group of disorders

1. An abnormal haemoglobin is synthesized – in which there is an amino acid substitution in either the α or β globin chain. Various different haemoglobins may occur. The most common is HbS, leading to sickle cell anaemia in which the RBC sickle when exposed to low oxygen tensions. *Homozygous* patients have *sickle disease* – severe haemolytic anaemia with sickle crises. *Heterozygotes* have *sickle cell trait* in which there is no anaemia but crises may occur with severe anoxia or infections, or both. Hb C, D and E are well recognized.
2. Reduced synthesis of normal globin chains – leads to α *or* β *thalassaemias*. The clinical picture varies according to the quantity of abnormal haemoglobin present and whether the patient is homo- or heterozygous. The red cells are more rigid and are destroyed in marrow or circulation.

Features of haemoglobin S, C, D and E disease

In order of frequency of prevalence

TABLE 8.4

Haemoglobin	World distribution	Anaemia		Quantity of abnormal haemoglobin (%)	Clinical features
HbS	Central Africa, Mediterranean, India	Mild to severe; target and sickle cells	Homozygotes	80–90	Severe haemolysis Growth impairment Sickle crises with tissue infarcts Leg ulcers
		None, few target cells	Heterozygotes	35	Severe hypoxia will induce crises
HbC	West Africa	Mild; many target cells	Homozygotes	90	Mild haemolysis
		None; few target cells	Heterozygotes	40	None
HbE	SE Asia	Mild; many target cells	Homozygotes	90	Mild haemolysis
		None	Heterozygotes	40	None
HbD	Indian continent	None; few target cells	Homozygotes	95	None
		None	Heterozygotes	40	None

Complications of sickle cell anaemia

1. Sickling crises – precipitated by infection, dehydration, low temperature
2. Aplastic crises – caused by papovavirus B19 infection
3. Infection

    i. Pneumococcal infections ⎱
    ii. Salmonella osteomyelitis ⎰ well recognized

4. Gall stone formation due to excessive bilirubin production
5. Chronic leg ulceration
6. Aseptic bone necrosis
7. Renal damage but not of major importance because of 1–3 above

Haematological features of α- and β-thalassaemia

TABLE 8.5

Diagnosis	Hb electrophoresis	Haemolytic anaemia
α-thalassaemias		
1. Gene deletion ⎱ trait ⎱	Normal	None
2. Gene deletion ⎰ ⎰		Mild
3. Gene deletion – HbH disease	HbH – 10–15 per cent	Moderate
4. Gene deletion – hydrops fetalis	Hb Bart's – 90 per cent	Fatal *in utero*
β-thalassaemias		
1. Homozygotes	HbF, HbA$_2$	Severe (major) or moderate (intermedia)
2. Heterozygotes	HbA$_2$, ± HbF	Mild (minor)

MCV, MCH reduced in all varieties, target cells and normoblasts in thalassaemia major

Aplastic anaemia

Pancytopenia (anaemia, leucopenia, thrombocytopenia) due to aplasia of the bone marrow; tend to present as infection, purpura or bleeding. Diagnosis is made by marrow biopsy: hypocellular.

PRIMARY

1. Idiopathic – up to 50 per cent of series
2. Congenital (Fanconi) – rare

SECONDARY

1. Drugs

 i. Dose-related – busulphan, 6-mercapto-
   purine, cyclophosphamide, chlorambucil,
   vinblastine, azathioprine
 ii. idiosyncratic – phenylbutazone, oxyphen-
   butazone, gold salts, chloramphenicol,
   sulphonamides, penicillamine

  only well
  recognized
  quoted;
  many others

2. Chemicals – benzene and many aromatic hydrocarbon solvents, insecticides, TNT, hair dyes

3. Ionizing – dose related radiations >10 Gy may prove irreversible

 i. accidental – radiology, radiotherapy, isotopes
 ii. therapeutic – bone marrow ablation

4. Infections – HBV, EBV, CMV, rubella

Poor prognostic features in aplastic anaemia

1. White blood count – <0.4 × $10^9/\ell$ (400/mm^3) for >2 weeks
2. Platelet count – <20 × $10^9/\ell$ (20 000/mm^3) for >2 weeks
3. Reticulocytes – <10 × $10^9/\ell$ (10 000/mm^3; <0.1 per cent)

Treatments of aplastic anaemia

1. Stop aetological agents if recognized
2. Supportive therapy

 i. transfusion of blood products
 ii. treatment of infection

Many patients with mild to moderate aplasia improve spontaneously. About 10 per cent with severe aplasia die in 1–2 years

3. Oxymethalone or lithium are usually ineffective in severe aplasia
4. Bone marrow transplant
5. Anti-thymocyte globulin or anti-lymphocyte globulin

may prove effective but both are complex, specialist proce-dures with a 40–50 per cent 5-year survival success rate

Neutrophil leucocytosis (Neutrophilia)

Count >10.0 × $10^9/\ell$ (10 000/mm^3)
Very frequently found. Often accompanying a fever.

1. Bacterial infections – especially generalized or local pyogenic bacteria; most common cause
2. Acute haemorrhage or haemolysis
3. Trauma, burns, surgery
4. Tissue necrosis – myocardial infarct, vasculitis
5. Disseminated solid tumours
6. Corticosteroid therapy
7. Myeloproliferative disease – CGL, polycythaemia, myelosclerosis
8. Metabolic diseases – diabetic coma, acute renal failure, gout, eclampsia
9. Physiological – neonates, pregnancy, exercise, stress

Leukaemoid reaction

Count >40.0 × $10^9/\ell$ (40 000/mm^3)

An excessive leucocytosis in which immature cells, pro-myelocytes or myelocytes, are found in the peripheral blood. Usually involves granulocytes. A leukaemoid reaction is distinguished from CGL (*see* page 125) by the presence of large numbers of mature neutrophils and few blasts; the LAP (*see* page 116) is high, the Philadelphia chromosome is absent and the spleen impalpable.

1. Acute severe infections – more common in splenectomized individuals and children
2. Advanced disseminated malignancy
3. Acute haemolysis

Leuco-erythroblastic anaemia

Erythroblasts together with primitive white cells in the peripheral blood.

1. Marrow infiltration by a malignancy – carcinoma, myeloma
2. Myelosclerosis – myeloid metaplasia
3. Myeloid leukaemias
4. Severe haemorrhage or haemolysis
5. Infection – TB or fungi
6. Granulomas – sarcoid, TB, histiocytosis X
7. Lipidoses ⎫ very rare
8. Marble bone disease ⎭

Neutropenia

Count <2.5 × $10^9/\ell$ (2500/mm³)

1. Infections
    i. viral
        (a) influenza
        (b) infectious mononucleosis (EBV)   } the most
        (c) infectious hepatitis   common causes
        (d) acute viral infections of childhood
    ii. bacterial
        (a) overwhelming septicaemia – particularly Gram-
            negative and staphylococcal
        (b) typhoid
        (c) brucellosis
2. Drug-induced – neutropenia tends to be prolonged
    i.   co-trimoxazole
    ii. phenytoin
    iii. carbimazole
    iv. tolbutamide   } marrow suppression
    v.   chlorpromazine
    vi. mepacrine
3. SLE or other collagen-vascular diseases
4. As part of general pancytopenia
    i. splenomegaly with or without portal hypertension
    ii. bone marrow failure
5. Benign – often in Africans; cyclical – rare
6. In association with severe folate deficiency

Eosinophilia

Count >0.4 × $10^9/\ell$ (400/mm³)

1. Drug allergy – penicillins and sulphonamides chiefly
2. Parasitic infestations – particularly those with a migratory life
   cycle
    i.   *Ascaris lumbricoides* – roundworm
    ii. *Taenia solium, T.saginata* – tapeworm
    iii. *Ancylostoma* – hookworm
    iv. *Toxocara canis, T.cati*
3. Allergic diseases
    i. bronchial asthma
    ii. hay fever

4. Skin disease
    i.   atopic eczema and urticaria
    ii. scabies
    iii. dermatitis herpetiformis
5. Hodgkin's disease or a carcinoma
6. Pulmonary eosinophilia – lung infiltrates
    i.   parasites passing through lungs – tropical eosinophilia
    ii. aspergillosis
    iii. polyarteritis nodosa
7. Hypereosinophilic syndrome – rare

Lymphocytosis

Count >3.5 × $10^9/\ell$ (3500/mm³)

1. Virus infections
    i.   infectious mononucleosis
    ii. viral infections of childhood
    iii. acute infectious lymphocytosis
2. Parasitic infestation – toxoplasmosis
3. Bacterial infections   *Bordetella*
    i.   brucellosis
    ii. tuberculosis
4. Chronic lymphocytic leukaemia

Monocytosis

Count >0.8 × $10^9/\ell$ (800/mm³) – infrequent

1. Infectious mononucleosis
2. Chronic bacterial infections
    i.   brucellosis
    ii. bacterial endocarditis
    iii. tuberculosis
3. Protozoan diseases
4. Monocytic leukaemia, Hodgkin's disease and occasionally carcinoma

Non-leukaemic myeloproliferative disorders

1. Polycythaemia vera
2. Essential thrombocythaemia
3. Myelosclerosis

Diagnosis of polycythaemia
TABLE 8.6

	Males	Females
Haemoglobin	>18.0 g/dl	>17.0 g/dl
Packed cell volume	>0.55	>0.47
Red cell count	>6.0 × $10^{12}/\ell$	>5.5 × $10^{12}/\ell$
Total red cell volume	>36 ml/kg	>32 ml/kg

See also Table 8.2, page 100

Causes of polycythaemia

PRIMARY

Polycythaemia vera – increase in red and white cells, also platelets

SECONDARY

Red cells only
1. Hypoxic
   i.   chronic lung disease with $\dot{V}/\dot{Q}$ imbalance – easily the most common
   ii. R to L shunts (cyanotic heart disease)
   iii. Obesity – Pickwickian syndrome
   iv. high altitude
   v.   central hypoventilation
2. Inappropriate erythropoietin
   i.   renal conditions
        (a) polycystic renal disease
        (b) hydronephrosis
        (c) post-transplant
        (d) hypernephroma
   ii. tumours
        (a) uterine fibromas
        (b) cerebellar haemangioblastoma
        (c) hepatocellular carcinoma
3. Overtransfusion
4. 'Blood doping'

RELATIVE

Contracted circulating volume
1. Plasma loss
   i.   burns
   ii. severe diarrhoeas
2. Dehydration – water depletion
3. 'Stress' or 'spurious' polycythaemia

Complications of polycythaemia

1. Thrombosis
2. Haemorrhage
3. Peptic ulcers
4. Myelofibrosis with marrow failure
5. Hyperuricaemia – in 25–30 per cent, of whom 5–10 per cent develop gout
6. Possible leukaemic transformation
7. Bruising easily – platelet dysfunction

Causes of a raised platelet count

1. Post-haemorrhage, operation or splenectomy
2. Chronic iron deficiency
3. Chronic infections
4. Malignancy
5. Rheumatoid arthritis
6. In some patients with polycythaemia vera, myelosclerosis and chronic granulocytic leukaemia
7. Essential thrombocythaemia – rare; count may reach $>1000 \times 10^9/\ell$

Leucocyte alkaline phosphatase

Low or undetectable in
1. Chronic granulocytic leukaemia
2. Paroxysmal nocturnal haemoglobinaemia
   HYPOPHOSPHATASIA
Raised in
1. Infections
2. Stress
3. Steroid therapy
4. Myelofibrosis
5. Polycythaemia vera
6. Chronic inflammation

Causes of splenomegaly

There are multiple causes which vary on a geographical basis.

EUROPE
1. Portal hypertension – the most common
2. Leukaemias
3. Malignant lymphomas
4. Myeloproliferative disorders
5. Haemolytic anaemias
6. Chronic infections
7. Storage diseases

GLOBALLY

1. Chronic parasitic infections, especially
   i.   malaria
   ii. leishmaniasis
   iii. schistosomiasis
2. Haemoglobinopathies
3. Portal hypertension
4. Tropical splenomegaly syndrome

Blood coagulation

Disorders of haemostasis

1. Acquired abnormalities
   i.   platelet defects
        (a) thrombocytopenia
        (b) drug-induced functional abnormalities
   ii. coagulation deficiencies
        (a) liver disease
        (b) anticoagulants
        (c) vitamin K deficiency
   iii. combined defects
        (a) intravascular coagulation
        (b) fibrinolysis
   iv. acquired anticoagulants
        (a) post-partum   ⎫ rare
        (b) lupus anticoagulant ⎭
2. Congenital coagulation deficiencies (haemophilia A is the most
   common clinically important congenital defect)
   i.   haemophilia A ⎫ sex-linked recessive ⎰ VII
   ii. haemophilia B ⎭ deficiency of factor ⎱ IX
   iii. von Willebrand's disease – abnormal platelets and plasma
        factors – rare
3. Inherited platelet abnormalities – rare conditions, present as
   menorrhagia

Causes of thrombocytopenia

The most common cause of bleeding

IMPAIRED PRODUCTION

1. Megakaryocyte depression
   i.   drugs
   ii. chemicals
   iii. viral infections

2. As part of general marrow failure
   i.   malignant infiltration of marrow
   ii. multiple myeloma
   iii. myelosclerosis
   iv. leukaemia
   v.   aplastic leukaemia
   vi. megaloblastic anaemia

ENHANCED DESTRUCTION

1. Immune causes – none common
   i.   drug-induced
   ii. SLE
   iii. chronic immune thrombocytopenia purpura (ITP)
   iv. autoimmune thrombocytopenic purpura
   v.   secondary immune thrombocytopenia
        (a) post-infection
        (b) CLL
        (c) lymphomas
2. Disseminated intravascular coagulation (DIC) – not uncommon

SEQUESTRATION OF PLATELETS – hypersplenism

DILUTIONAL LOSS – massive transfusion of old blood

Laboratory diagnosis of platelet disorders

Blood count

Thrombocytopenia   Normal platelet count

1. Bone marrow – failure of   1. Bleeding time-acquired defects
   marrow
2. Screen for DIC   2. Platelet aggregation studies
3. Platelet antibodies – drug-   with
   induced conditions
                                    i.   ADP ⎤ measured by
                                    ii. adrenalin ⎥ light transmission
                                    iii. collagen ⎥ through a suspension of platelets
                                    iv. ristocetin ⎦

                                 3. Adhesion tests
                                 4. Factor VIII clotting assay –
                                    in case of von Willebrand's
                                    disease

Coagulation cascade and fibrinolytic pathways

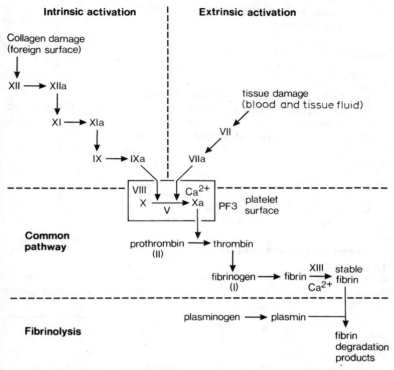

Figure 8.1 Coagulation cascade and fibrinolytic pathways. Intrinsic system: injury to endothelium exposes collagen and other components that activate factor XII. Extrinsic system: tissue damage liberates lipoproteins which activate factor VII. PF3: exposed on platelet surface after aggregation – a phospholipid. (1 mole XIa amplifies to 2×10^8 mole fibrin)

Haemostasis involves

1. Vascular constriction diminishing blood flow
2. Platelet plug formation
3. Local blood coagulation

Coagulation factors

FIBRINOGEN GROUP

Factors I, V, VIII, XII

 i. activity lost during coagulation – not present in serum

ii. increased in inflammation, pregnancy and oral contraception
iii. V and VIII store poorly
iv. liver synthesis

PROTHROMBIN GROUP

Factors II, VII, IX, X

i. liver cell synthesis – vitamin K needed
ii. not consumed during coagulation (except for II) – present in serum
iii. preserved in stored plasma

CONTACT GROUP

Factors XI, XII

i. not vitamin K dependent
ii. store well in plasma

Acquired coagulation deficiencies
TABLE 8.7

Condition	Platelet count	APTT	PT	TT	FDP	Coagulation factors
DIC	↓	↑	↑	↑	↓	I ↓
Liver disease	N or ↓	↑	↑	N	N or ↑	VIII ↑
Vitamin K deficiency	N	↑	↑	N	N	II VII IX X ↓
Acquired anticoagulant	N	↑	↑ or N	N	N	Variable
Heparin	N	↑	↑	↑	N	N

APTT = activated partial prothrombin time, PT = prothrombin time, TT = thrombin time, FDP = fibrin degeneration products, N = normal, ↑ = increased, ↓ = decreased.

Laboratory tests for diagnosis of coagulation disorders
TABLE 8.8

Test	Function	Normal range
Prothrombin time (PT)	Extrinsic and common pathways	12–14 seconds
Activated partial thromboplastin time (APTT)	Intrinsic and common pathways	30–40 seconds
Thrombin time (TT)	Fibrinogen → fibrin conversion	10–12 seconds

Disseminated intravascular coagulation (DIC) ('Consumption coagulopathy')

The features of DIC depend upon the rapidity and magnitude of the coagulation stimulus. If there is endothelial damage or tissue damage or platelet aggregation, coagulation factors and platelets are consumed with fibrin deposition.

DIC ranges from a fulminant haemorrhagic syndrome (gross depletion) to a mild form neither recognized nor of consequence (no depletion of coagulation factors).

Conditions associated with DIC

1. Infection – the most important group of causes
   i.   Gram-negative septicaemia
   ii. meningococcal infection
   iii. staphylococcal infection
   iv. falciparum malaria
2. Trauma and surgery – often with infection or burns
3. Obstetric – unusual, but severe
   i.   premature placental separation
   ii. amniotic fluid embolus
   iii. retained placenta
   iv. eclampsia
4. Liver disease
   i.   advanced cirrhosis
   ii. fulminant liver failure
5. Malignancy – usually a laboratory diagnosis only
   i.   mucin-secreting carcinoma
   ii. promyeloentic leukaemia
   iii. prostatic carcinoma
6. Miscellaneous
   i.   incompatible blood transfusion
   ii. snake venom
   iii. anaphylaxis
   iv. hypoxia
   v.   hypothermia

Diagnosis of DIC

1. Minor changes – increase in fibrin/FDP
2. More advanced changes

    i.   thrombocytopenia

    ii. PT   ⎫

    iii. APTT ⎬ times prolonged

    iv. blood film shows

       (a) microangiopathic haemolytic anaemia

       (b) fragmented red cells

3. At worst, whole blood may not clot due to fibrinogen consumption. No platelets on blood film, coagulation factors consumed, mortality 100 per cent

Complications of blood transfusion

TABLE 8.9

Early	Late
1. Haemolytic reactions – mismatched transfusion	1. Transmission of
2. Allergic reactions to white cells	i. hepatitis A; B; non-A non-B
3. Pyrogenic reactions to HLA antibodies anti-IgA antibodies	ii. malaria iii. cytomegalovirus and EBV
4. Circulatory overload	iv. AIDS
5. Clotting abnormalities after multiple units of blood	v. syphilis – rare
6. Hyperkalaemia in chronic renal failure	2. Iron overload – after 100 units 3. Sensitization to Rhesus D antigen

Blood viscosity

$$\text{Viscosity} = \frac{\text{Shear stress}}{\text{Shear rate}} \quad \begin{array}{l}\text{(force applied to the liquid)}\\ \text{(resulting flow rate)}\end{array}$$

Clinical conditions of raised viscosity

The majority depend upon raised haematocrit and raised ESR

1. Serum abnormalities

    i.   increased fibrinogen

    ii. macroglobulinaemia

    iii. myeloma

2. Red cell concentration

    i.   polycythaemia vera

    ii. secondary polycythaemia

3. Red cell shape
   i.   sickle cell disease
   ii. spherocytosis
4. Miscellaneous
   i.   postoperative venous thrombosis
   ii. dehydration
   iii. hypovolaemic shock
   iv. diabetes mellitus
   iv. malignancy

Erythrocyte sedimentation rate (ESR)

Raised in a wide number of conditions as a non-specific index of organic disease. Sedementation depends upon

1. The difference in specific gravity between erythrocytes and plasma
2. The rate at which red cells clump
3. The rate at which red cells form rouleaux

   i.   fibrinogen ⎫
   ii. α_2-and γ-globulin ⎬ concentrations

The ESR is low in dehydration, polycythaemia and HbSS – in HbSS rouleaux do not form

how – effective syndrome

Haematological disease causing cerebral infarction

1. Sickle cell disease
2. Polycythaemia rubra vera
3. Leukaemia
4. Thrombotic thrombocytopenia purpura
5. Hyperviscosity syndromes
6. Essential thrombocythaemia

(>100) & high –

① Myeloma
② Temp Arteritis
③ Polymyalgia Rheumatica
④ SLE
⑤ Carcinoma
⑥ Chronic Infection

Chapter 9
Medical oncology

Leukaemias

Classification

TABLE 9.1

Acute	Chronic

Myeloblastic (AML)
M0 Undifferentiated (AUL)
M1 Myeloblastic, poorly differentiated (AUL)
M2 Myeloblastic (AML)
M3 Promyelocytic (AProL)
M4 Myelomonoblastic (AMML)
M5 Monoblastic (AMoL)
M6 Erythroleukaemia (EL)
	Granulocytic (CGL or CML)
	Lymphocytic (CLL) – mostly B-cells
	Less common varieties
	  i. hairy-cell leukaemia
	  ii. dysmyelopoietic syndromes

Lymphoblastic (ALL) non-T, non-B – common Thy-ALL B-cell ALL – rare	

In children – 85 per cent of cases are of the ALL type, most of the remainder being AML.
In adults – AML is most common. Prognosis of AML worse than ALL.
CLL is more common than CGL.
Both occur in middle aged to elderly.
70 per cent of CGL changes to an acute leukaemia.
In CLL terminal marrow failure occurs. Mean prognosis of both is 3–5 years.

Comparison of CGL and CLL

TABLE 9.2

CLINICAL FEATURES	CGL	CLL
Anaemia	Present	Present
Systemic features	Weight loss, anorexia, fever	
Peripheral nodes	Normal	Enlarged in most Tonsils in some
Splenomegaly	Often massive	Enlarged
Skin	Normal	Pruritus in many. Zoster
Median survival	3–4 years	3–5 years
LABORATORY FEATURES		
Leucocytosis	$50–500 \times 10^9/\ell$ All forms of myeloid cells found in peripheral blood	$30–300 \times 10^9/\ell$ 70–99 per cent peripheral cells appear as mature lymphocytes
Philadelphia chromosome	Present	Absent
Bone marrow	Hypercellular with granulocytic predominance	Lymphocytic replacement
Neutrophil alkaline phosphatase score	Low	–
Anaemia	Normochromic, normocytic	Normochromic, normocytic
Platelets	Raised, normal or reduced	Reduced
Serum immunoglobulins	Normal	Reduced with advanced disease
Serum B_{12}	Raised and B_{12} binding capacity increased	Normal
Treatment	Busulphan	Chlorambucil or cyclophosphamide

Differentiation between leukaemoid reactions and chronic granulocytic leukaemia

TABLE 9.3

	Leukaemoid reaction	CGL
Mature polymorphs	Predominate	Suppressed
Myeloblasts	Unusual	May be >80 per cent of total WBC
Leucocyte alkaline phosphatase score	High	Low
Philadelphia chromosome	Absent	Present
Spleen	Impalpable	Almost invariably enlarged

Malignant lymphomas

Three types
1. Hodgkin's disease
2. Non-Hodgkin's lymphoma
3. Burkitt's lymphoma – Epstein–Barr (E-B) virus associated

Hodgkin's disease

Definition
A chronic lymphoproliferative disorder of unknown aetology with distinctive features. Fatal if untreated. Importance:
1. Among the commonest malignancies in young adults
2. Cure possible in most cases

Features
1. Painless enlarging nodes in neck, axillae, groin or mediastinum
2. Most common between ages of 15 and 30 years, men >women
3. Fever, night sweats, weight loss, pruritus – old patients
4. Pain with consumption of ethanol
5. No single test diagnostic save for biopsy

Histological classification (Rye nomenclature)

TABLE 9.4

Morphology	Prognosis	
Lymphocytic predominance	Good	Most common in children, mostly boys
Nodular sclerosis		Most frequent, chiefly women
Mixed cellularity		Second most frequent, chiefly males
Lymphocytic depletion	Poor	Infrequent

Staging of Hodgkin's disease and non-Hodgkin's lymphoma

TABLE 9.5

Stage	Features
I	Disease limited to a single region
II	Two or more regions on same side of diaphragm or disease at an extra-lymphatic site and one or more nodal areas above or below the diaphragm
III	Nodes involved both sides of the diaphragm together with extra-lymphatic site, or spleen or both
IV	Disseminated disease with or without lymph node enlargement

In Hodgkin's disease, patients are sub-classified A or B indicating the absence or presence respectively of systemic symptoms.

Non-Hodgkin's lymphomas

TABLE 9.6 Classification

Nodular	Prognosis
1. Lymphocytic, well differentiated – rare	Favourable
2. Lymphocytic, poorly differentiated – most common	Favourable
3. Histiocytic	Unfavourable
4. Mixed forms	Unfavourable
Diffuse	
More common in patients <35 or >65 years	
1. Lymphocytic, well differentiated – similar to CLL	Favourable
2. Lymphocytic, poorly differentiated – common	Unfavourable
3. Histiocytic	Unfavourable
4. Mixed	
5. Burkitt's	

CLINICAL FEATURES

1. Median age at presentation – 50 years, males >females
2. Painless asymmetrical enlargement of lymph nodes
3. Constitutional symptoms less common than in Hodgkin's
4. Liver, spleen and retroperitoneal node involvement common
5. Waldeyer's ring involved in 10 per cent
6. Skin, brain or gut involvement not infrequent
7. More common than Hodgkin's disease; accounts for 3 per cent of all cancers
8. Chlorambucil remains the drug of choice

HAEMATOLOGICAL FEATURES

1. Anaemia – normochromic, normocytic, autoimmune haemolytic at times
2. Late features – neutropenia, thrombocytopenia or leucoerythroblastic anaemia
3. Lymphosarcoma cells in peripheral blood of some patients
4. Focal marrow involvement in 20 per cent of cases

IMMUNOLOGICAL FEATURES

1. Majority are monoclonal B-cell tumours
2. Occasional monoclonal paraprotein – IgG or M
3. In children the disease may be thymic in origin

Multiple myeloma

A malignancy of B lymphocytes. Diagnosis depends upon the presence of at least two of the following features

1. Monoclonal paraprotein in serum and urine
2. Neoplastic plasma cells in bone marrow
3. Lytic bone lesions

MYELOMA PROTEIN ABNORMALITIES

1. Immunoglobulin types
   i.   IgG paraprotein – 65 per cent ⎫
   ii. IgA paraprotein – 32 per cent ⎬ of patients
   iii. IgM, D or mixed – 3 per cent   ⎭
2. Concentration of normal serum immunoglobulins depressed
3. Bence-Jones protein (free-light chains) in 66 per cent of cases

CLINICAL FEATURES

1. Bone pain, pathological fractures
2. Anaemia, abnormal bleeding tendency
3. Repeated infections
4. Renal failure and symptoms related to hyercalcaemia
5. Amyloid features – usually sub-clinical
6. Hyperviscosity syndrome – infrequent, usually IgM myeloma

FACTORS ASSOCIATED WITH A POOR PROGNOSIS

Median survival is 2 years with a 20 per cent 4-year survival

1. Plasma urea >13 mmol/ℓ at presentation – median survival 2 months
2. Hb <8.0 g/dl
3. Serum albumin <30 g/ℓ
4. Bence–Jones proteinuria >200 mg/dl

CAUSES OF RENAL FAILURE IN MYELOMA

1. Casts of Bence-Jones protein in tubules – irreversible
2. Hypercalcaemia nephropathy – should be reversible
3. Amyloid – arterioles, glomeruli; irreversible
4. Urate nephropathy – iatrogenic
5. Recurrent renal infection – immune paresis of myeloma

CAUSES OF A PARAPROTEIN

1. Benign monoclonal gammopathy ⎫
2. Multiple myeloma   ⎬ the most common
3. Macroglobulinaemia   ⎭
4. Malignant lymphoma and CLL

BENIGN AND MALIGNANT PARAPROTEINS

TABLE 9.7

Serum features	Malignant	Benign
Immunoglobulin fragments	Present	Absent
Suppression of normal immunoglobulins	Always	Rarely
Serum concentration of 10 g/ℓ or more	Almost invariably	Very infrequently
Progressive rise in paraprotein concentration	Always	Very rarely

FEATURES OF HYPERVISCOSITY SYNDROME

Usually an IgM paraprotein

1. Weakness
2. Confusion, coma
3. Blindness – specific retinopathy
4. Congestive heart failure
5. Serum viscosity >4 cp – normal 1.5–1.8 cp, low shear rate

Tumour lysis syndrome

DEFINITION

Metabolic effects of rapid destruction of tumour cells by intensive cytotoxic chemotherapy. Primarily concerns patients with bulky, highly chemosensitive undifferentiated lymphomas, acute lymphoblastic lymphoma and Burkitt's lymphoma.

FEATURES

1. Hyperkalaemia
2. Hyperphosphataemia – tumour breakdown
3. Hypocalcaemia
4. Hyperuricaemia – usually >1.2 mmol/ℓ
5. Raised creatinine and plasma urea

All features are worsened if there is renal impairment before treatment is commenced.

Indications for platelet transfusion

1. Excessive bleeding – platelet count $<20 \times 10^9/\ell$
2. Counts $<10 \times 10^9/\ell$ without bleeding
3. DIC – but short survival of platelets
4. Idiopathic thrombocytopenic purpura
5. Post-removal of very large spleens

Indications for granulocyte transfusion

1. Neutropenia of $<0.5 \times 10^9/\ell$ with infection (10^{10} granulocytes needed daily)
2. During early days following marrow grafts

Indications for bone marrow transplant

1. Severe aplastic anaemia and persistent severe granulocytopenia or thrombocytopenia
2. Acute leukaemia – childhood ALL, AML and poor prognosis ALL in remission
3. Chronic granulocytic leukaemia in chronic phase or in blast crisis
4. Combined immunodeficiency
5. Inherited red cell defects such as thalassaemia (selected patients)

Metabolic complications of malignancy

1. Hypercalcaemia – see page 68
2. Hyponatraemia – see page 66
3. Hypokalaemia – not common

   i.   metabolic or respiratory alkalosis
   ii. increased urine loss – Cushing's or ectopic ACTH
   iii. excessive gut loss – villous adenoma, VIPoma, Zollinger–Ellison syndrome

4. Acute renal failure – not common

   i.   obstruction by tumours of prostate, bladder, pelvis or retroperitoneum
   ii. hypercalcaemia
   iii. hyperuricaemia
   iv. intra-renal myeloma paraprotein deposition
   v.   infiltration of kidney by lymphoma

vi. tumour lysis syndrome – *see* page 129
vii. over-use of gentamicin – not infrequent
viii. cytotoxic drugs: cisplatin, streptozotocin
5. Tumour lysis syndrome – *see* page 129
6. Hypomagnesaemia

Neurological complications of malignancy

1. Brain metastasis – about 25 per cent of intracranial tumours
   Most frequently from bronchus, breast, kidney, gut or ovary.
   Over half of patients have multiple lesions. Hemispheres,
   cerebellum and brain stem most frequently involved
2. Vertebral column and spinal cord metastases
   A vertebral metastasis is most commonly secondary to a
   tumour of bronchus, breast, prostate or kidney. Prostate and
   breast cancers often produce multiple deposits usually in the
   thoracic spine. Cord metastases are rare
3. Carcinomatous meningitis
   Occurs most often in patients with leukaemias or lymphomas.
   The major carcinomatous origins are breast, bronchus or
   stomach. Diffuse and nodular meningeal infiltration occurs. II,
   V and VI nerves most frequently affected. Papilloedema
   common
4. Non-metastatic syndromes

   i.   encephalopathic syndrome – temporal lobes, brain stem or
        cord
   ii. cerebellar degeneration – depletion of Purkinje cells; limb
        and gait ataxia, nystagmus
   iii. sensory neuropathy – destruction of dorsal root ganglia
   iv. mixed neuropathy – uncommon
   v.   myasthenic (Eaton–Lambert) syndrome – bronchial
        tumours: myopathy with limb pain
   vi. dermatomyositis – usually associated with cancer of lung,
        breast or ovary

5. CNS infection

   i.   herpes zoster
   ii. *Cryptococcus neoformans* } in patients with lymphoma
   iii. progressive multifocal leucoencephalopathy – most often
        found in patients with advanced Hodgkin's and is
        secondary to a papovavirus invasion

6. Iatrogenic neurological disease
    i. radiation damage
        (a) brain – especially after treatment of paranasal sinuses
        (b) cord
        (c) nerves
    ii. anti-neoplastic drugs
        (a) vincristine – peripheral neuropathy
        (b) encephalopathy – L-asparaginase ⎱ rare
        (b) cerebellar damage – 5-fluorouracil ⎰

Miscellaneous complications of malignancy

1. Haematological
    i.   anaemia – blood loss, infection, infiltration of bone marrow, renal impairment, haemolysis
    ii. pancytopenia – extensive marrow replacement, typically in breast, lung and prostate cancer and non-Hodgkin's lymphoma
    iii. thrombocytopenia – secondary to chemotherapy, hypersplenism or DIC which may complicate any cancer with a propensity to widespread metastasis
    iv. bleeding –
        (a) local as from ulcerating cancer or perforation of vessel
        (b) clotting impaired secondary to platelet deficiency or impaired coagulation from liver failure

2. Abdominal
    i.   ascites – common complication of advanced gut tumours and may be a presenting feature of ovarian cancer or abdominal lymphoma; also occurs in metastatic breast carcinoma
    ii. bowel obstruction – major complication either directly due to tumour or to adhesions
    iii. intestinal obstruction – acute or subacute varieties common in many patients with advanced cancers
    iv. inflammatory complications – oesophagitis, gastritis, pancreatitis, cholecystitis and acute liver distension may all occur
    v.   bleeding – most likely to be intraluminal
    vi. urological complications – consist chiefly of haemorrhage, obstruction and infection

3. Pulmonary and cardiac

i. pleural effusion – may occur in any metastic malignancy but most common in breast, ovarian, lung cancer and lymphomata. Exudates. *See also* page 39

ii. lung metastasis – discrete and usually multiple rounded secondaries often complicate breast, gut, thyroid and renal carcinomata, sarcomas and germ cell tumours in children; lymphangitis carcinomatosa occurs most frequently in women with breast cancer

iii. infection, radiation pneumonitis and LVF have to be separated; *Pneumocystis carinii* may complicate lymphomas

iv. Pulmonary thromboembolism is quite common in patients with abdominal or pelvic cancers

v. Pericardial effusion – occurs in a small proportion of patients with lung cancer

vi. Stridor – mediastinal masses, lymphoma of neck and thyroid cancer are all implicated

vii. SVC obstruction – carcinoma of the lung is the most common cause

4. Pathological fractures

Chapter 10

Gastroenterology

Gingival hyperplasia

1. Pregnancy (especially second trimester)
2. Oral contraceptive pill
3. Acute leukaemia – quite common
4. Neutropenia
5. Phenytoin
6. Cyclosporin
7. Tuberous sclerosis

Causes of oral pigmentation

1. Post-trauma or inflammation – common
2. Racial – Negro, East Asian and Asian
3. Fixed drug eruptions – pigmentation and blisters
4. Keratosis (leucoplakia) and candidosis
5. Peutz–Jegher's syndrome – mouth, lips and peri-oral region
6. Addison's disease – gums, and inner surface of lips } rare
7. Acanthosis nigricans – often in mouth
8. Blue line on gums from Hg, bismuth or Ag poisoning

Causes of impairment of taste

1. Smoking
2. Chronic nasal blockage
3. Dentures
4. Drugs

    i.   levodopa
    ii. captopril
    iii. metronidazole
    iv. penicillamine
    v. lithium carbonate
    vi. griseofulvin

5. Hypothyroidism
6. Depressive illness
7. Advancing years
8. Temporal lobe epilepsy

Loss of taste (ageusia)

Often difficult to reach a diagnosis.

1. Local X-irradiation
2. Inflammatory disease of buccal cavity
3. Lesions of chorda tympani may cause unilateral loss of taste in the anterior two-thirds of the tongue

Nausea

CAUSES

1. Stomach
   i.   gastritis – food, alcohol, drugs
   ii. ulcers
   iii. rapid bleeding
   iv. carcinoma
   v.   pyloric stenosis
2. Acute surgical abdominal conditions
3. Pregnancy – first trimester
4. Metabolic
   i.   diabetic pre-coma
   ii. hypercalcaemia
   iii. chronic renal failure – urea >50 mmol/ℓ (300 mg/100 ml)
5. Severe pain or anxiety
6. CNS
   i.   migraine
   ii. drugs
   iii. raised intracranial pressure
   iv. Menière's disease
   v.   psychogenic
7. Acute infections
   i.   urinary tract
   ii. pneumonia
   iii. viral hepatitis
   iv. pertussis
8. Infants and children – *see* pages 198 and 201

Causes of acute upper gastro-intestinal bleeding

1. Common
    i. duodenal ulcer ⎱ main causes
    ii. gastric ulcer   ⎰
    iii. stress ulcers
    iv. acute erosions
    v. Mallory–Weiss tear
    vi. gastritis and duodenitis
2. Uncommon
    i. oesophageal ulcer
    ii. oesophageal varices
    iii. gastric cancer
    iv. anastomotic ulcer
    v. anticoagulant therapy
    vi. bleeding disorders
    vii. aortic aneurism
3. Rare
    i.   hereditary haemorrhagic telangiectasia
    ii. pseudoxanthoma elasticum
    iii. pancreatic bleeding

Vomiting

Causes may include

1. Severe pain
2. Early pregnancy
3. Gastric irritants
    i.   alcohol
    ii. many different drugs
    iii. ulcers
4. Advanced chronic renal failure – urea >50 mmol/ℓ (300 mg/100 ml)
5. Hypercalcaemia – Ca^{2+} >3.5 mmol/ℓ (14 mg/100 ml)
6. Neurological
    i.   migraine
    ii. vestibular dysfunction
    iii. increased intracranial pressure
    iv. autonomic neuropathy
7. Psychogenic and anxiety

Causes of dysphagia

1. Hold up of food in chest
    i.   carcinoma of oesophagus or cardia ⎤
    ii. oesophageal stricture   ⎥
    iii. mediastinal neoplasm   ⎬ mechanical
    iv. aortic aneurysm – infrequent   ⎥
    v.   foreign body   ⎦
    vi. achalasia – uncommon   ⎤
    vii. systemic sclerosis – rare   ⎥
    viii.diffuse muscle spasm – older patients ⎬ muscular
    xi. Chagas' disease – S. America   ⎦

2. Pain on swallowing
    i.   oesophagitis – peptic, monilial (common)
    ii. achalasia
    iii. diffuse muscle spasm
    iv. carcinoma

3. Difficulty in swallowing
    i.   infected throat – most common
    ii. functional
    iii. XI nerve lesions   ⎤
    iv. motor neuron disease ⎦ rare

4. Choking and regurgitation
    i.   bilateral hemiplegia ⎤ bilateral upper motor
    ii. multiple sclerosis   ⎦ neuron lesions
    iii. motor neuron disease ⎤ lower motor ⎤
    iv. polyneuropathy   ⎬ neuron   ⎥
    v.   syringomyelia   ⎦ lesions   ⎬ rare
    vi. dystrophia myotonica   ⎥
    vii. myasthenia gravis   ⎦

5. Lump in throat
    i.   pharyngeal pouch
    ii. thyroid enlargement
    iii. post-cricoid carcinoma
    iv. globus hystericus

Precipitating factors in gastro-oesophageal reflux

1. Hiatus hernia
2. Pregnancy

3. Surgical procedures
   i.   vagotomy
   ii. partial gastrectomy
4. Infancy and old age
5. Progressive systemic sclerosis

Peptic ulcer

TABLE 10.1

	Gastric	*Duodenal*
Site	Middle of lesser curve	Duodenal bulb
Pathology	Benign or malignant	Benign
Pain and vomiting	Periods of freedom and relapse	
Weight loss and anorexia	Suggest malignancy	
Frequency		2–3 times more than gastric ulcer
Social class	Both common in poor people	
H$^+$ ions	Normal quantities, biliary reflux	⅓ hyperchlorhydric
Blood group	O is commonest	
Sex	Equal distribution	

Antacids

1. Aluminium hydroxide – constipation
2. Magnesium trisilicate – diarrhoea
3. Calcium carbonate – hypercalcaemia; dose-dependent

Indications for gastric surgery

1. Perforation
2. Persistent bleeding
3. Malignancy
4. Pyloric stenosis

Complications of gastric surgery

MECHANICAL

1. Dumping syndrome
2. Vomiting or regurgitation – in up to 25 per cent of patients
3. Diarrhoea – quite common

NUTRITIONAL

All late (years) developments. The more the stomach has been removed the more likely is a complication.

1. Weight loss
2. Iron deficiency anaemia – quite common
3. B_{12} deficiency anaemia – always after total gastrectomy
4. Folic acid deficiency – to a minor degree
5. Osteomalacia – 5–10 per cent of patients. Vitamin D malabsorption
6. Osteoporosis – calcium malabsorption
7. Pulmonary tuberculosis – chance of infection increased

Gastric neoplasms

There are no characteristic symptoms of any of these tumours. If spread has occurred preoperatively then cure cannot be expected.

1. Adenocarcinoma – the third most common tumour in UK. Poor prognosis. Suggestive features
   i.   indigestion with anorexia or weight loss
   ii. vomiting with pyloric or lower oesophageal obstruction
   iii. gastric ulcer responding poorly to treatment
   iv. dyspepsia and weight loss a few years after gastric surgery
   v.   irregular liver or supraclavicular nodes
2. Lymphoma ⎤
3. Gastric polyps ⎬ rare
4. Leiomyomas ⎦

Gastric electrolytes

TABLE 10.2

Ion	Parietal cell (mmol/ℓ)	Non-parietal cell (mmol/ℓ)
H^+	160	–
Na^+	–	160
Cl^-	170	125
K^+	10	10
HCO_3^-	–	45

Causes of haematemesis and melaena

1. Chronic DU – 30–40 per cent ⎤
2. Chronic GU – 10–20 per cent ⎟
3. Acute erosions – 20–30 per cent ⎟
4. Mallory–Weiss – 10–15 per cent ⎬ of different series
5. Gastric cancer – 2–5 per cent ⎟
6. Portal hypertension – 2–5 per cent ⎟
7. Unexplained – 5–10 per cent ⎦

Causes of lower gut bleeding

1. Haemorrhoids and anal fissure – common
2. Carcinoma of rectum or colon
3. Diverticulitis
4. Inflammatory bowel disease
5. Angiodysplasia – elderly
6. Infective diarrhoea – amoebic or bacillary dysentery
7. Pseudomembranous colitis – after a course of an antibiotic
8. Irradiation proctitis
9. 'Gay bowel' syndrome
10. May complicate NSAIDs
11. Unexplained

Absorptive sites of the small bowel

PROXIMAL

1. Products of digestion of fat, carbohydrate and protein
2. Iron
3. Folic acid
4. Fat and water soluble vitamins

TERMINAL ILEUM

1. Vitamin B_{12}
2. Bile salts

Small gut flora

The concentrations of aerobic and anaerobic bacteria increase with increasing distance down the small gut.

Nutritional effects
1. Advantageous – synthesis of folate and vitamin K
2. Deleterious – deconjugation of bile salts and ingesting nutrients

Assessment of small gut function

1. Serum or plasma concentrations of
   i.   iron
   ii. folate
   iii. B_{12}
   iv. albumin and calcium
   v.   potassium
   vi. amino acids

2. Fat absorption – measurement of stool fat over 4–5 days. If excretion is more than 7 per cent of intake an abnormality is present. However, fat absorption may be normal in the presence of severe small gut disease
3. Carbohydrate absorption
   i. urinary xylose excretion – abnormal result in coeliac disease and tropical sprue. Invalid if renal failure present
   ii. lactose tolerance test. Positive if blood glucose concentration rises only a little after an oral load of lactose
   iii. glucose tolerance test. A diabetic curve in patient with steatorrhoea suggests a pancreatic cause
4. Function of terminal ileum – Schilling test. Urinary radioactivity as a measure of B_{12} absorption. Normally >7 per cent of dose excreted in 24 hours
5. Bacterial overgrowth
   i. sampling of jejunal contents for culture
   ii. urinary indican concentration – raised in the presence of abnormal small gut flora. Reduced in pancreatic steatorrhoea
   iii. ^{14}C bile salt breath test (^{14}C-glycocholic acid) – expired ^{14}C after an oral dose is a measure of bacterial bile-salt deconjugation

Gut peptides

There are many endocrine cells within the mucosa of the gastrointestinal tract. The hormones produced control different aspects of digestion. A number of rare endocrine syndromes are associated with overproduction of some of these hormones.

1. Gastrin – from G cells of antral mucosa in response to distension or protein
2. Pancreatic polypeptide – secreted when the pancreas is stimulated and thus induces negative feedback control
3. Cholecystokinin – secreted in upper small gut in response to protein or fat
4. Gastric inhibitory polypeptide – released by the presence of carbohydrate to stimulate insulin secretion
5. Secretin – from duodenum in response to H^+ leading to a flow of alkaline fluid from pancreas
6. Motilin – continuously secreted by small gut aiding emptying
7. Neurotensin – from lower small gut in response to carbohydrate or fat. Reduced gastric H^+ production and increased pancreatic bicarbonate secretion

8. Enteroglucagon – released by lower small gut and colon in the presence of fat or carbohydrate. Promotes mucosal growth, enhancing absorption

Causes of malabsorption

GROSS STRUCTURAL LESIONS

1. Gastric surgery – the most common, but mild
2. Inflammatory bowel disease
3. Following intestinal resection
4. Bacterial overgrowth in
   i.   blind loops – afferent loop stasis
   ii. diverticulae
5. Giardiasis following gastric surgery
6. Fistulae – malignant or Crohn's
7. Diabetic autonomic neuropathy
8. Arterial insufficiency – infrequent
9. Progressive systemic sclerosis – rare
10. Amyloidosis – rare

INFECTION

1. Acute enteritis – short-term malabsorption
2. Traveller's diarrhoea – common
3. Parasitic infestation – *Giardia lamblia* is the most frequent – common
4. Tuberculosis – secondary to active TB, usually in immigrants

MUCOSAL LESIONS

1. Gluten-sensitive enteropathy – fairly common; (coeliac disease)
2. Tropical sprue – very common tropical disease
3. Mesenteric vascular disease
4. Whipple's disease ⎫ very rare
5. Intestinal lymphangiectasis ⎭
6. Hypogammaglobulinaemia and abetalipoproteinaemia – rare

DRUG CAUSES

The most common

1. Alcohol – may interfere with absorption and exacerbate dietary defects
2. Neomycin – mucosal damage, increase in bile salt loss
3. Cholestyramine – bile salt binding

MALDIGESTION

1. Parenchymal liver disease ⎫
2. Obstructive jaundice   ⎬ deficiency of bile salts
3. Alcoholic liver disease – impaired pancreatic function
4. Zollinger–Ellison syndrome – rare; profuse diarrhoea

NON-GUT DISEASES

1. Thyrotoxicosis – common
2. Dermatitis herpetiformis – overlaps with coeliac disease
3. Malignant disease
4. Collagen – vascular diseases

Causes of malabsorption leading to malnutrition

TABLE 10.3

Disease	Main deficiencies – weight loss in all
Post-gastrectomy	Iron, B_{12}
Coeliac disease	Iron, folic acid
Pancreatic disease	Fat soluble substances – vitamins A, D, K
Crohn's disease	Iron, B_{12}, K^+, Mg^{2+}
Stagnant bowel syndromes	B_{12}

Causes of subtotal villous atrophy (as shown by jejunal biopsy)

1. Coeliac disease
2. Disaccharidase deficiency
3. Dermatitis herpetiformis
4. Tropical sprue (not invariably)
5. Zollinger–Ellison syndrome

Individuals at risk of malnutrition

1. Elderly living alone
2. Expectant mothers
3. Alcoholics
4. Mentally ill
5. Immigrant children
6. Post-total gastrectomy

Clinical features of advanced malabsorption

1. Shrivelled and pale
2. Atrophic tongue
3. Abdomen distended by dilated oedematous gut
4. Dry skin, ecchymoses on forearms
5. Finger clubbing
6. Dependent oedema
7. Peripheral neuropathy
8. Tetany easily provoked
9. Waddling gait of osteomalacia
10. Bulky, fatty, rancid stools (>20 g fat daily)

Major diarrhoea-causing diseases

Diarrhoea is scientifically defined as the passage of stools weighing >200 g/day. Clinically diarrhoea is a change in bowel habit with frequent evacuation of stools which have a consistency different from normal.

1. Infective diarrhoea – the most common world-wide
2. Carcinoma of colon
3. Thyrotoxicosis
4. Malabsorption leading to steatorrhoea
5. Crohn's disease
6. Ulcerative colitis and proctitis
7. Anxiety – acute and chronic
8. Irritable bowel syndrome
9. Diabetes mellitus – autonomic neuropathy
10. Iatrogenic
    i.   drugs; *see* list below
    ii. post-vagotomy
    iii. small bowel resection

Drug causes of diarrhoea

1. Oral (or parenteral) broad-spectrum antibiotics
2. Magnesium trisilicate or cimetidine
3. Iron preparations
4. Indomethacin and other NSAIDs
5. Methyldopa or propanolol
6. Theophylline
7. Methotrexate
8. Levodopa

Differential features of three gut diseases

TABLE 10.4

	Ulcerative colitis	Crohn's disease	Coeliac disease
Clinical features			
Bloody diarrhoea	Common	Infrequent	Not present
Abdominal pain	Often	Frequent	Uncommon
Perianal disease	Infrequent	60–70%	Not a feature
Signs of malabsorption	Never	Frequent	Always
Abdominal mass	Rare	Frequent	Not present
Iritis	Transient	Occurs	Not a feature
Fever	May occur	Frequent	Uncommon
Investigations			
Anaemia	Iron	Iron and B_{12}	Iron and folate
ESR	Raised	Raised	Normal
Iron absorption	Normal	Normal	Abnormal
B_{12} absorption	Variable	Abnormal	Normal
Radiology			
Rectal involvement	Always	Infrequent	Not present
Distribution	Continuous	Discontinuous 'Skip-lesions'	Often continuous
Mucosa	Fine ulceration	'Cobblestones'	Smooth with flocculation and fragmentation
Strictures	Rare	Common	Absent
Fistulae	Very rare	Occur	Absent
Pre-Disposition to Neoplastic change	20–30 times greater chance of adenocarcinoma	None	Increased risk of small bowel reticulum cell sarcoma

Ulcerative colitis and Crohn's disease are collectively known as inflammatory bowel disease. After duodenal ulcer, Crohn's disease is the second most common cause of small bowel ulceration.

Radiological features of ulcerative colitis

INACTIVE DISEASE

1. Fine mucosal granularity with thick outline
2. Mucosal ulcers
3. Mucosal islands
4. Pseudopolyps
5. Dilatation (toxic megacolon; barium enema should not be performed at this stage)
6. Dilated ileum
7. Narrow rectum with increased sacrorectal space (>1 cm)

INACTIVE CHRONIC DISEASE

1. Loss of haustra
2. Narrow shortened bowel
3. Benign stricture
4. Malignant stricture or raised surface of an adenocarcinoma

Extra-intestinal features of inflammatory bowel disease

1. Sacro-iliitis – 20 per cent
2. Ankylosing spondylitis – 5 per cent
3. Aphthous ulcers – 20 per cent
4. Transient large joint arthropathy – 10 per cent
5. Erythema nodosum – 10 per cent
6. Eye conditions – up to 10 per cent

    i.   conjunctivitis
    ii. episcleritis
    iii. uveitis

7. Liver disease – *see* page 162 – 5 per cent
8. Pyoderma gangrenosum – 1 per cent
9. Renal – oxalate stones (page 94)

Main causes of the surgical acute abdomen

1. Inflammation

    i.   acute appendicitis
    ii. salpingitis
    iii. sigmoid diverticulitis
    iv. acute cholecystitis
    v.   pancreatitis

2. Perforation

    i.   duodenal ulcer
    ii. gastric ulcer
    iii. traumatic rupture of a viscus

3. Obstruction

    i.   biliary stone
    ii. ureteric stone
    iii. tumour of large bowel
    iv. small gut adhesions
    v.   strangulated hernia
    vi. strangulation of small gut

4. Haemorrhage
   i. ruptured ectopic pregnancy
   ii. traumatic rupture of spleen
   iii. ruptured ovarian follicle
5. Torsion
   i. ovarian cyst
   ii. testis
6. Vascular
   i. leaking aortic aneurysm
   ii. dissecting aneurysm
   iii. mesenteric vascular occlusion
7. Extra-abdominal
   i. acute chest infection ⎫
   ii. pleurisy   ⎬ medical
   iii. myocardial infarct ⎪
   iv. herpes zoster   ⎭
8. Munchausen's syndrome

Medical causes of acute abdominal pain

 1. Diabetic ketoacidosis (gastric dilatation)
 2. Acute pyelonephritis
 3. Migraine
 4. Acute gastritis
 5. Henoch–Schönlein purpura
 6. Hypercalcaemia
 7. Sickle-cell crises
 8. Intestinal parasites ⎫
 9. Porphyria   ⎬ rare
10. Lead poisoning   ⎭
11. Tabes dorsalis – increasing incidence

Main causes of chronic constipation

Constipation considered to be present if a patient evacuates <3 times weekly or passes <30 g of stool per day

1. Painful anal lesions
2. 'Lazy' bowel
3. Metabolic and endocrine
   i. pregnancy – very common
   ii. diabetes mellitus

iii. hypothyroidism – quite common
iv. hypercalcaemia – less common
v. hypokalaemia
4. Prolonged bed rest ⎫ may be related
5. Poor roughage intake ⎭
6. Colonic cancer
7. Depression
8. Dyschezia
9. Spastic colon
10. Neurological abnormalities
  i. autonomic neuropathy – diabetes the most common cause
  ii. Hirschsprung's disease ⎫ quite uncommon
  iii. adult megacolon ⎭
11. Opiates, aluminium hydroxide, antidepressants, anticho-
linergies, anti-parkinsonism agents, anticonvulsants

Causes of incontinence of faeces

PARTIAL OR INADVERTENT INCONTINENCE

1. Severe diarrhoea
2. Carcinoma of rectum
3. Rectal prolapse
4. Following local surgery – temporary
5. Severely ill or disorientated

COMPLETE INCONTINENCE

1. Neurological
  i. multiple sclerosis – impaction or neuromuscular loss
  ii. cauda equina lesion – LMN lesion
2. Traumatic – damage to the puborectalis sling
  i. surgery
  ii. accidental injury
3. Idiopathic – the largest group

Intestinal worms

NEMATODES (round worms)

1. *Ascaris lumbricoides* (round worm) – Far East, tropical Africa,
South East Europe, Central and S. America
2. *Trichuris trichiura* (whipworm) – most tropical areas
3. *Ancylostoma duodenale* or *necator americanus* (hookworm) –
tropics and sub-tropics. Very common

4. *Strongyloides stercoralis* – Far East, East and West Africa, South America. Lungs, duodenum and jejunum
5. *Enterobius vermicularis* (threadworm) – Tropics, Europe and USA

CESTODES (tapeworms)

1. *Taenia saginata* – Middle East and tropical Africa. Beef
2. *Taenia solium* – similar distribution. Larval stage called cysticercosis. Pork
3. *Diphyllobothrium latum* (fish tapeworm) – Scandinavia, parts of Africa, Middle and Far East, northern American and USSR
4. *Hymenolepis nana* (dwarf tapeworm) – virtually all tropical areas
5. *Dipylidium caninum* – worldwide distribution, small gut

Bacterial food poisoning

TABLE 10.5

Organism	Food involved	Pathogenesis	Incubation period (hours)
Staphylococcus aureus	Salads, milk containing foods	Enterotoxins A to E	1–6
Clostridium perfringens	Faecal contamination, spores survive cooking. Cooked meals, pies, stews	Ingestion of living organism	12–24
Salmonella spp	Contaminated meat–poultry, pork, ham, beef	Mucosal invasion	12–48
Bacillus cereus	Fried rice	Mucosal invasion	1–6
C.botulinum	Preserved or canned foods	Spores producing a heat-labile neurotoxin	12–36

Radio-opacities on plain abdominal X-ray

1. Tablets
2. Phleboliths
3. Calcified lymph nodes – in patients >50 years
4. Gall stones
5. Aorta, splenic and iliac arteries
6. Renal stones and calcification

7. Fetus
8. Calcified costal cartilages
9. Calcified fibroids
10. Calcification in pancreas or adrenal gland ⎫
11. Cysticerci   ⎬ rare
12. Dermoids – bone or teeth   ⎭

Chapter 11
Liver, biliary tree and pancreas

Classification of jaundice

TABLE 11.1

Parenchymal liver disease – cholestasis		Urine findings

1. Hepatitis
   i. viral
   ii. autoimmune		

2. Alcoholic hepatitis		Bilirubin
3. Cirrhosis		
4. Drugs and toxins		
5. Venous obstruction – rare		

Extra-hepatic		

1. Gall stones in biliary tree
2. Pancreas
   i. carcinoma
   ii. pancreatitis
3. Biliary tree stricture – less
   common
	90 per cent of all cases of surgical jaundice. Pale stools, dark urine	Bilirubin
		No urobilinogen
		if complete
		obstruction

Non-hepatic – unconjugated hyperbilirubinaemia	

1. Haemolysis
   i. neonatal – physiological; one-third of all births
   ii. acquired – *see page 105*
	Excess
	urobilinogen

2. Familial unconjugated hyperbilirubinaemias – Gilbert's; most common; *see also page 154*	

Diagnostic steps in a patient with jaundice

TABLE 11.2

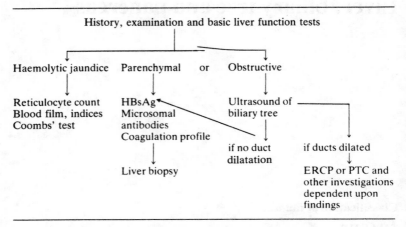

Ultrasound examination of the biliary tree demonstrates obstruction in up to 95 per cent of cases. If doubt exists then CAT scan of the liver will show dilated intrahepatic ducts

Jaundice in relation to age at presentation

TABLE 11.3

Age (years)	Likely causes
15–20	Acute viral hepatitis – the majority Chronic active hepatitis Gilbert's syndrome (5 per cent) Haemolysis
40–50	Alcoholic liver disease – 50 per cent
>70	Extra-hepatic biliary obstruction

Liver biopsy

Liver biopsy should always be preceded by an ultrasound examination.

INDICATIONS

1. Morphological diagnosis of acute and chronic jaundice and sequelae of acute hepatitis

2. Diagnosis of secondary deposits of tumours
3. Diagnosis of systemic disease – sarcoid, reticuloses, storage diseases
4. Drug induced liver injury
5. Unexplained abnormalities of liver function
6. Investigation of some patients with PUO
7. Hepatomegaly: fatty liver, cirrhosis, neoplasia or amyloid may be diagnosed

CONTRAINDICATIONS

1. Coagulation disorders
2. Obstructive jaundice
3. Prominent ascites
4. Uncooperative patient
5. Hydatid disease

COMPLICATIONS

1. Haemorrhage
2. Bile peritonitis – usually self-limiting
3. Puncture of incorrect tissue – lung, kidney, bowel, gall bladder, pancreas

Investigation of obstructive jaundice

TABLE 11.4

	Transhepatic cholangiography (PTC)	Endoscopic retrograde cholangio-pancreatography (ERCP)
Risk to patient	Small but real	Less
Cost	Cheap	Expensive equipment
Expertise required	Little	Considerable
Success	99 per cent with dilated intrahepatic ducts. Up to 70 per cent with normal ducts	Up to 90 per cent
Contra-indications	Coagulation defects	Acute pancreatitis
Advantages	Demonstration of biliary duct lesions	Demonstration of pancreatic duct disease
Complications	Bile peritonitis Haemorrhage	Acute pancreatitis

Hyperbilirubinaemia with normal liver function tests

UNCONJUGATED

1. Haemolytic anaemia
2. Neonatal jaundice – *see* page 220
3. Glucyronyl transferase deficiency

   i. Gilbert's syndrome
   ii. Crigler–Najjar syndrome

CONJUGATED

1. Systemic conditions (LFTs may be abnormal)

   i. Atrial fibrillation with pulmonary emboli
   ii. Heart failure
   iii. Infection – septicaemia or pneumonia
   iv. Cholestasis in Hodgkin's disease
   v. Post-cardiopulmonary bypass

2. Familial – rare

   i. Dublin–Johnson syndrome
   ii. Rotor's syndrome

Causes of post-operative jaundice

1. Transfusion of virus hepatitis
   i. B or non-A non-B
   ii. E-B virus   ⎱ especially when fresh blood is used
   iii. cytomegalovirus   ⎰ such as to supply clotting factors
2. Sepsis
3. Trauma
4. Biliary tree damage
5. Halothane hepatitis
6. Mismatched transfusion

Antibiotic-induced jaundice

Acute hepatic cholestasis, chronic active hepatitis or hepatic necrosis – usually associated with fever, rash, eosinophilia, or eosinophilic infiltration of the liver biopsy

1. Isoniazid
2. Pyrazinamide
3. Sulphonamides

4. Nitrofurantoin
5. Erythromycin
6. Tetracycline
7. Chloramphenicol

Aetiology of ascites of hepatic origin

Number of complex processes in combination

1. Portal hypertension
2. Serum albumin <30 g/ℓ; liver cell impairment
3. Hyperaldosteronism; >330 pmol/ℓ following 2
4. Sodium and water retention – consequent upon 3
5. Reduction in GFR – aggravating 4

Causes of ascites

1. Malignant disease – common
   i. peritoneal secondary deposits
   ii. IVC obstruction
2. Nephrotic syndrome – children
3. Pancreatic disease
4. Constrictive pericarditis
5. Tuberculous peritonitis
6. Chylous – lymphatic obstruction; rare
7. Mesothelioma   } Extrahepatic
8. Vascular – rare
   i. hepatic vein thrombosis
       (a) idiopathic
       (b) malignancy related
       (c) veno-occlusive
   ii. portal vein thrombosis
       (a) abdominal
       (b) umbilical

Hepatic – cirrhosis; common. Results from abnormalities of sodium metabolism and local factors affecting fluid exchange at the level of the mesenteric capillary and hepatic sinusoid (*see* above)

Examination of ascitic fluid

TABLE 11.5

Appearance	Clear or yellow/green	Hepatic origin
	Bloody	Suggestive of malignancy
	Turbid/white	Infected, chylous or malignancy
Cell count	$0-0.3 \times 10^9/\ell$ mononuclear	Sterile ascites
	$>0.5 \times 10^9/\ell$ neutrophils	Bacterial infection
	Chiefly mononuclear	Possibly tuberculous
Protein	$<25\,g/\ell$	Uncomplicated cirrhosis Transudate
	$>30\,g/\ell$	Exudate, inflammatory

It is usually necessary to have ascitic fluid cultured for bacteria and AAFB and also examined for malignant cells. Protein concentrations of ascitic fluid may not be diagnostically reliable. With successful diuretic therapy protein concentration of ascitic fluid tends to rise.

Complications of ascites

1. Pressure effects
   i.   inguinal hernias
   ii. splinting of diaphragm
   iii. basal lung collapse
2. Spontaneous bacterial peritonitis–mortality 70–90 per cent because it tends to be misdiagnosed

Acute hepatitis

The most common liver disease in the world. Many attacks are sub-clinical.

CAUSES

1. Hepatitis A virus (HAV) – infectious hepatitis; most infections occur in children
2. Hepatitis B virus (HBV) – serum hepatitis
3. Non-A non-B hepatitis
4. Hepatitis D (delta) virus (HDV)
5. Cytomegalovirus (CMV) – infants and the immunosuppressed
6. Infectious mononucleosis due to EB virus – morphologically in almost all, clinically in half
7. Herpes simplex virus
8. Coxsackie virus
9. Measles
10. Varicella zoster

TROPICAL VIRUSES

1. Yellow fever
2. Lassa fever
3. Marburg virus
4. Ebola fever
5. Rift valley fever

Sources of viral hepatitis

1. Via transfusion of blood or blood products
2. Heterosexual or homosexual promiscuity
3. Intravenous drug abuse
4. Direct contact with patients with hepatitis
5. From food or fluids in countries with poor hygiene and where hepatitis is common
6. Tattooing

Comparisons between the major hepatitides

TABLE 11.6

	Hepatitis A	Hepatitis B	Non-A non-B
Incubation period	2–6 weeks	2–6 months	6 weeks – 3 months
Route of transmission	Faecal – oral	Venereal, salivary, or via blood products	Parenteral – commonest post-transfusion hepatitis
Virus detectable in	Faeces	Blood	
Diagnosis	Serum antibody	Antigen in serum and tissues	Unknown
Prophylaxis	γ-globulin	Hyperimmune globulin. Vaccination	
Chronic sequelae	No	Yes	Yes

HDV is an incomplete small virus which can only exist in the presence of HBV infections. Occurs either simultaneously with an HBV infection or in a HBV carrier. Most common in drug addicts and homosexuals. The infection is more severe than that of HBV; may be fulminant. Carriers of HBV and HDV are likely to develop cirrhosis.

Hepatitis B serology

1. Surface antigen HBsAg leading to HBsAb (antiHBsAg)
2. Core antigen in Dane particles HBcAg – may not be infective
3. e antigen – HBeAg. Considered to be very infectious

serology   Ag   s ⇒) e ⇒) c   Ab   c ⇒) e ⇒) s

Possible sequelae of an acute hepatitis

1. Direct recovery
2. Post-hepatitis syndrome – months ⎱ health
3. Temporary relapse
4. Chronic persistent hepatitis ⎱
5. Chronic aggressive hepatitis leading to cirrhosis – possible death

5 per cent of patients with hepatitis B; perhaps more with non-A non-B

6. Fulminant hepatitis – rapid ⎱ death
7. Sub-acute hepatic nerosis – months ⎰
8. Asymptomatic carrier state – HBsAg positive for remainder of life – almost 5 per cent of patients

Chronic hepatitis

An inflammatory reaction in the liver continuing without improvement for at least six months.

Three main forms

1. Chronic persistent hepatitis – nearly always self-limiting
2. Chronic lobular hepatitis – variable, some progress to cirrhosis
3. Chronic aggressive hepatitis – may well progress to cirrhosis

They are diagnosed by liver biopsy and not by clinical or biochemical features.

TABLE 11.7

Morphology	Chronic persistent	Chronic lobular	Chronic aggressive
Portal inflammation	Present	Present	Present
Periportal inflammation	Absent	Minimal	Present
Piecemeal necrosis	Absent	Scattered	Present
Bridging necrosis	Absent	Absent	Often present
Fibrosis	Minimal	In some	Prominent

Causes of chronic hepatitis
TABLE 11.8

Chronic persistent	Chronic aggressive
1. HBV	1. HBsAg
2. Non-A non-B	2. Non-A non-B
3. Autoimmune in some	3. Alcohol
4. Drugs	4. Drugs
i. aspirin	i. oxyphenisatin
ii. isoniazid	ii. to v. as for chronic persistent
iii. methyldopa	5. Chronic active hepatitis – immune
iv. paracetamol	serology positive
v. cytotoxics	6. Wilson's disease – serum copper and
5. Inflammatory bowel disease	caeroloplasmin
6. Idiopathic	7. α_1 antitrypsin deficiency – serum and antitrypsin concentration
	8. Haemochromatosis – serum iron, IBC
	9. Primary biliary cirrhosis – mitochondrial antibodies
	10. Idiopathic – (up to 25 per cent of series)

Chronic active hepatitis (Auto-immune hepatitis)
CLINICAL FEATURES

1. Females of 10–25 and 50–65
2. Mimics acute viral hepatitis
3. Responds to steroids
4. Extra-hepatic features

  i. arthralgia
  ii. spider naevi and palmar erythema
  iii. amenorrhoea } common
  iv. acne
  v. rashes – occasionally
  vi. thyroid, pleura, eyes, pericardium, arthritis, vasculitis, ulcerative colitis, Coombs' positive anaemia, leucopenia or fibrosing alveolitis – very occasionally)

SEROLOGY

1. Characterized by high titres of antibodies to nuclear, smooth muscle, liver mitrochondrial microsomal antigens
2. DNA binding positive
3. High serum IgG and to a lesser extent IgM and A
4. Coombs' positive anaemia
5. Strong association with HLA – B8, DW3

Alcoholic liver disease (ALD)

OCCUPATIONAL RISKS OF ALCOHOLIC CIRRHOSIS INCREASED IN

1. Company directors and executives
2. Licensed traders
3. Entertainers and those who entertain as part of their occupation
4. Servicemen
5. Doctors and their wives
6. Waiters
7. Brewers

VARIETIES OF ALCOHOL-INDUCED LIVER DISEASE

1. Fatty liver – without features or causes hepatomegaly
2. Alcoholic hepatitis – florid spider naevi, liver enlarged
3. Micro- or macronodular cirrhosis
4. The above changes with cholestasis or siderosis, or both
5. Chronic active hepatitis
6. Central sclerosing hyaline necrosis
7. Hepatoma in 15–25 per cent of cirrhotics

Major metabolic effects of ethanol

1. Hepatic gluconeogenesis $\downarrow$, leading to hypoglycaemia
2. Albumin and transferrin synthesis $\downarrow$
3. Lipoprotein synthesis $\uparrow$ especially VLDL
4. Fatty acids accumulate
5. Ketoacidosis
6. Serum triglycerides $\uparrow$
7. Fatty liver due to decreased fatty acid oxidation
8. Lactate production $\uparrow$, leading to hyperuricaemia
9. Blood and tissue acetaldehyde $\uparrow$
10. Catecholamine release $\uparrow$

Primary biliary cirrhosis

Uncommon disease of middle aged women, clinically and biochemically mimicking obstructive jaundice. Characteristic liver histology. Overlap with scleroderma, CRST, Sjögren's, RA, SLE and RTA.

CLINICAL FEATURES	Incidence (%)
1. Female	90
2. Pruritus	80
3. Enlarged liver	80
4. Jaundiced	60
5. Pale stools, dark urine	60
6. Splenomegaly	50
7. Pigmentation	25
8. Xanthelasma	25
9. Ascites	15
10. Bone pain	5

INVESTIGATIONS	Incidence (%)
1. Alkaline phosphatase	100
2. Liver enzymes	80
3. Bilirubin	85
4. Liver copper	80
5. Cholesterol	80
6. Mitochondrial antibody – virtually excludes extra-hepatic obstruction	95
7. IgM raised	75
8. Antinuclear antibody	20

Wilson's disease (hepato-lenticular degeneration)

Gradual accumulation of copper in liver and basal ganglia. Rare disease. Treatable with penicillamine.

CLINICAL FEATURES

1. Presents in teenagers
2. Liver features
3. Tremor, rigidity, dysarthria, impairment of intellect
4. Kayser–Fleischer rings

AUT REC

BIOCHEMICAL DIAGNOSTIC FEATURES

1. Caeruloplasmin – reduced
2. Serum copper – reduced
3. Urine copper – raised
4. Liver copper – raised

Haemochromatosis

Iron overload
Gross increase in total iron stores – usually not more than 1.5 g in men – to 100 g. Serum transferrin oversaturated; serum ferritin much raised.

CAUSES

Primary (idiopathic) haemochromatosis – autosomal recessive
Secondary iron overload

1. Complicating multiple transfusions ⎫
   i. thalassaemia   ⎬ by far the most
   ii. sickle-cell anaemia   ⎪ common causes
2. Complicating alcoholic cirrhosis   ⎭
3. Post-portocaval anastomoses
4. Dietary excess – Bantu siderosis (cooking pots)

TABLE 11.9 Comparison of primary and secondary forms

Feature	Primary	Secondary
Family history	Present	None
Alcohol abuse	No	Common
Pigmentation	⎱ Very constant	
Cardiac involvement	⎰ features	Infrequent
Arthropathy		
Degree of iron excess	Marked	Moderate
Predisposition to hepatoma	Much increased	Increased
HLA	A3, B14	No association

Liver complications of inflammatory bowel disease

BILIARY

1. Pericholangitis – in about 5 per cent of patients
2. Bile duct carcinoma
3. Gall stones

HEPATO-CELLULAR

1. Chronic aggressive hepatitis – 2 per cent
2. Cirrhosis – 3 per cent
3. Fatty change – 6 per cent
4. Amyloid – 1 per cent
5. Granulomata
6. Abscesses

Causes of fatty infiltration of the liver

Common histological finding but non-specific of any particular disease

1. Obesity – very common
2. Starvation, malnutrition and malabsorption
3. Alcohol – both following a 'binge' or in addicts
4. Diabetes – when out of control
5. Many systemic illnesses – self-resolving
6. Parenteral nutrition
7. Drugs – especially i.v. tetracycline and corticosteroids
8. Pregnancy – common
9. Reye's syndrome

Causes of hepatomegaly

1. Fatty infiltration
2. Malignancy

    i.   secondary tumours
    ii. chronic granulocytic leukaemia

3. Acute alcoholic hepatitis
4. Venous congestion

    i.   right heart failure
    ii. constructive pericarditis
    iii. tricuspid stenosis   ⎫
    iv. Budd–Chiari syndrome ⎬ rare

5. Infectious causes

    i.   hepatitis A, B, non-A non-B
    ii. herpes simplex and yellow fever
    iii. secondary syphilis
    iv. leptospirosis

6. Congenital

    i.   polycystic disease
    ii. Reidel's lobe

7. Storage disorders

Causes of hepatic granulomas

Collections of mononuclear cells which form multi-nucleate giant cells. The granulomas *per se* are asymptomatic

1. Tuberculosis $\Big\}$ the most common
2. Sarcoidosis
3. Crohn's disease
4. Primary biliary cirrhosis – in around 30 per cent of cases
5. Lymphoma and Hodgkin's disease
6. Toxins – beryllium; light bulb manufacture
7. Infections
8. Idiopathic – 25 per cent
9. Visceral leishmaniasis (with systemic features)

Portal hypertension

Present when the portal vein pressure is about 20 mmHg; the normal pressure is about 5–10 mmHg. Leads to gastro-oesophageal varices or ascites or both.

PRE-SINUSOIDAL – The portal vein 'end' of the liver. Liver function is relatively unimpaired and liver failure common.

1. Extra-hepatic portal vein obstruction
    i.   sepsis especially following exchange transfusion in neonates
    ii. hypercoagulable blood
    iii. pressure upon portal vein by carcinoma or lymphomas
2. Intra-hepatic portal vein obstruction
    i.   schistosomiasis – common in endemic areas
    ii. reticuloendothelial malignant infiltration of liver
    iii. sarcoidosis
    iv. primary biliary cirrhosis

SINUSOIDAL OR INTRAHEPATIC – liver failure and variceal bleeding not uncommon. Any advanced cirrhosis

POST-SINUSOIDAL – the hepatic vein 'end' of the liver
    i.   hepatic vein occlusion – Budd–Chiari syndrome
    ii. veno-occlusive (bush tea) disease

Causes of liver failure

TABLE 11.10

Chronic – gradual destruction	Acute – massive necrosis of liver cells

Cirrhosis
Chronic aggressive hepatitis
	Drugs
	  i. paracetamol overdose – the most
	     common cause
	  ii. halothane, mortality 80% ⎫
	              ⎬ idiosyncratic
	  iii. isoniazid ⎭
	
	Viral hepatitis
	  i. non-A non-B –
	     most common – 10% survival rate
	  ii. HAV – 33% – 45% survival rate
	  iii. HBV – 25% – 20% survival rate
	
	Toxins
	  i. carbon tetrachloride
	  ii. *Amanita phalloides*

Clinical features	
Bleeding tendency Stigmata of chronic liver disease Ascites very frequently Porto-systemic encephalopathy Renal impairment – 40%	May have early, severe abdominal pain No signs of chronic liver disease Variable jaundice Variable impairment of mental state Ascites not prominent Renal functional impairment in 50% Small liver – if present implies a bad prognosis

Acute on chronic liver failure

Precipitating causes

1. Bleeding
    i.   protein load via gut – varices, peptic ulcer
    ii. hypotension – underperfusion of liver
2. Protein load – dietary
3. Hypokalaemia – diuretics
4. Surgery
5. Opiates – reduced hepatic clearance
6. Infection – in any organ of the body

Prognostic criteria for successful portacaval shunt surgery

Shunt procedures are now used when variceal sclerosis has failed

1. Age <40 years
2. No jaundice
3. No ascites
4. No previous hepatic encephalopathy
5. Serum albumin >30 g/ℓ (3.0 g/100 ml)
6. Absence of alcoholic liver disease
7. No need for high IQ for subsequent occupation

Gall stones

PATHOLOGICAL TYPES

1. Solitary cholesterol – 95 per cent cholesterol ⎫
2. Bilirubin – very little cholesterol ⎬ 20 per cent of all – both types radiolucent
⎭
3. Mixed – calcium, bile pigments, cholesterol – 70–80 per cent of cases; radiopaque

AETIOLOGY

1. Abnormal bile salt metabolism – reduced trihydroxy bile acids
2. Increased liver synthesis of cholesterol
3. Oral contraceptives or oestrogens increasing liver cholesterol
4. Excess bilirubin – chronic haemolytic anaemias
5. Dietary factors
   i   predisposition in those taking a low fibre, high energy, high refined carbohydrate diet
   ii. half a bottle of wine daily appears to protect against cholesterol stones

TYPES OF PATIENTS DEVELOPING GALL STONES

1. About 15 per cent of the population
2. No evidence that obesity is causal
3. Equal prevalence in fair and dark coloured people
4. No relationship with high parity
5. Prevalence increases with age
6. Common in men and women

COMPLICATIONS OF GALL STONES

1. Remain in gall bladder and cause no symptoms – 50 per cent
2. Biliary colic
3. Obstructive jaundice
4. Ascending cholangitis
5. Pancreatitis
6. 5 per cent found by accident

Hepatic tumours

PRIMARY BENIGN

Uncommon

1. Cavernous haemangioma
2. Hepatocellular adenoma – appear to be related to oral contraception

PRIMARY MALIGNANT

Uncommon

1. Hepatocellular – hepatoma – close association with persistent HBV infection; α-fetoprotein raised in up to 75 per cent of patients
2. Cholangiocarcinoma – 20 per cent of primary liver cancers
3. Angiosarcoma – associated with vinyl chloride exposure

SECONDARY MALIGNANT

Common

1. Carcinoma – the most common; presages a poor prognosis
2. Lymphoma
3. Carcinoid – has to have metastasized to the liver to produce the carcinoid syndrome

Indications for liver transplantation

Age – post-puberty to <55 years

1. Primary hepatocellular carcinoma or cholangiocarcinoma
2. Primary biliary cirrhosis
3. Chronic active hepatitis

4. Budd–Chiari syndrome
5. Alcoholic cirrhosis
6. Biliary atresia

Aetiology of some tropical liver diseases

TABLE 11.11

Disease	Aetiology
1. Amoebic liver abcess	*Entamoeba histolytica* ⎫
2. Malaria; tropical splenomegaly syndrome	*Plasmodium* ⎬ protozoa
3. Schistosomiasis	*Schistosoma mansoni* and *japonicum* – trematodes
4. Hydatid disease	*Echinococcus granulosus* – cestode
5. Yellow fever	Arbovirus ⎫ viruses
6. Lassa fever	Arenavirus ⎭
7. Aflatoxicosis, hepatocellular carcinoma	*Aspergillus flavus* ⎫ malnutrition
8. Childhood cirrhosis	*Senecio* and *Crotalaria* spp ⎭ and hepatotoxins

Acute pancreatitis

CAUSES

1. Many idiopathic
2. Associated with gall stones and cholecystitis ⎫ majority
3. Alcoholism ⎭ of patients
4. Surgery to pancreas, biliary tree or stomach
5. Metabolic
   i.   hypercalcaemia
   ii. hyperlipidaemia (Fredericksen's type V>I>IV)

6. Drugs
   i.   oral contraceptives
   ii. corticosteroids

7. Viruses
   i.   mumps
   ii. Coxsackie virus group B

8. Miscellaneous
   i.   terminal chronic renal failure
   ii. hypothermia
   iii. trauma
   iv. pregnancy
   v.   acute liver failure

LABORATORY FEATURES

1. Leucocytosis
2. Raised serum or urinary amylase – raised in 80 per cent but is non-specific
3. Hyperglycaemia – early days – in 30–70 per cent
4. Hypocalcaemia – at days 4–8 – associated with a poor prognosis
5. Raised liver enzymes and bilirubin – obstructive, related to calculous disease of the biliary tree
6. Hyperlipidaemia – may occur as a result of, or proceed and be the 'cause' of, acute pancreatitis
7. Raised creatinine and urea – ARF in up to 20 per cent of patients
8. Coagulation disorders

Glucose
LDH
Urea
Calcium
Age
Glob   Alb
O2
Neut

Chronic pancreatitis

CAUSES

1. Alcoholism
2. Malnutrition in tropics
3. Gall stones – not a clear relationship
4. Unknown in many patients

FEATURES

1. Pain and weight loss
2. Malabsorption
3. Diabetes
4. Mild jaundice

Chapter 12

Endocrinology

The pituitary gland

Anterior pituitary hypersecretion

1. Giantism in children
2. Acromegaly in adults ⎫ rare
3. Cushing's disease ⎬
4. Hyperprolactinaemia ⎭

Acromegaly

Caused by an eosinophilic adenoma producing an excess of growth hormone.

CLINICAL FEATURES

1. Face – greasy skin, prognathism, large tongue, splayed teeth
2. Feet and hands – become broad and spatulate
3. CVS – hypertension, enlarged heart
4. Bones – overgrowth around joints leading to degenerative joint disease
5. Muscles – fibres hypertrophy but strength poor
6. Metabolic – 40 per cent glucose intolerance; 50 per cent hypercalciuria; 5 per cent hypercalcaemia (an overlap with hyperparathyroidism); hyperthyroidism in a few
7. Visual fields – compression of optic chiasma, nerves or tracts

OUTLOOK

Mortality rate increased by a factor of two. Deaths from hypertension and diabetes.

Cushing's disease

Hypersecretion of ACTH by basophil cells or chromophobe cells. Clinical features as for Cushing's syndrome – *see* page 179.

Hyperprolactinaemia

Many chromophobe tumours secrete prolactin. This is the commonest hormone-producing pituitary tumour.

CLINICAL FEATURES

Gonads become insensitive to gonadotrophins; thus in

1. Women – infertility and amenorrhoea. Galactorrhoea in up to 50 per cent
2. Men – infertility and impotence. Gynaecomastia occasionally

CAUSES OF HYPERPROLACTINAEMIA

1. Physiological
   i.   stress
   ii. pregnancy
   iii. breast-feeding

2. Drug-induced
   i.   oestrogens – including oral contraceptive pill
   ii. alpha methyldopa, reserpine – dopamine depletion
   iii. phenothiazines ⎫
   iv. metoclopramide ⎭ dopamine receptor blocking

3. Pathological
   i.   chronic renal failure
   ii. hypothalamic lesions
        (a) encephalitis
        (b) basal meningitis
        (c) trauma
        (d) sarcoid
   iii. pituitary tumour
        (a) prolactin secreting
        (b) growth hormone secreting
        (c) 'non-functioning' chromophobe adenoma
   iv. primary hypothyroidism

4. Chest wall – neural mediation
   i.   nipple stimulation
   ii. post herpes zoster (of T5)

Anterior pituitary hyposecretion

IN CHILDREN

1. Dwarfism – stunted growth ⎫ rare, caused by
2. Infantilism – subnormal ⎬ pituitary tumours.
   sexual development ⎭ Some idiopathic

DIFFERENTIAL DIAGNOSIS

1. Genetically small
2. Chronic disease
   i.   coeliac disease
   ii. chronic renal failure
   iii. congenital heart disease
3. Hypothyroidism
4. Turner's syndrome
5. Achondroplasia

IN ADULTS

Rare

CAUSES OF HYPOPITUITARISM

1. Tumours
   i.   chromophobe adenoma – the most common cause
   ii. suprasellar tumours
2. Trauma
   i.   accidental
   ii. surgical removal
   iii. previous X-irradiation
3. Granulomas
   i.   sarcoid
   ii. tuberculosis
   iii. histocytosis
4. Post-partum haemorrhage – Sheehan's syndrome

Cranial (neurogenic) diabetes insipidus

Failure of ADH production. Rare. Constant thirst, persistent excretion of hyposmolar urine.

CAUSES

1. Idiopathic
2. Acquired
    i.   trauma with rupture of the pituitary stalk
    ii. tumours in or around the pituitary (secondary or primary)
    iii. infectious – basal meningitis, abcess or encephalitis
    iv. iatrogenic – surgery, yttrium-90 implantation, irradiation
    v.   granulomas – sarcoid, tuberculosis or eosinophilic granu-
         loma
    vi. vascular – infarction of the pituitary (Sheehan's syndrome)
3. Familial – dominant or recessive inheritance – very rare
4. As a complication of steroid treatment of panhypopituitarism

DIAGNOSIS

1. Diuresis continues when fluid is withheld
2. Polyuria and thirst cease following i.m. desmopressin
3. There may be clinical and biochemical features of anterior
   pituitary failure also

The thyroid

Tests of thyroid function

1. Serum thyroxine – T4 } secreted by thyroid, almost
2. Serum tri-iodothyronine – T3 } entirely carried bound to thyroxine binding globulin and
   albumin. Apart from tissue
   effects the serum concentrations of T4 and T3 have a
   negative feedback on TSH
   secretion
3. Basal serum TSH
4. TRH–TSH test – normal response is shown by TSH
   concentrations increasing 1–30 mU/ℓ 20 minutes after 200 µg of
   i.v. TRH

SELECTION OF TESTS

This is generally straightforward, but note that
1. Acutely ill patients often have abnormal TFTs which become
   normal when the illness resolves

2. In geriatric practice the best indicator of thyroid status is basal TSH or TRH–TSH test
3. Pregnancy or the oral contraceptive pill raise serum concentrations of T4 and T3
4. Iodine, lithium, propanolol, phenytoin and salicylate } lower concentrations of T4 and T3

Hyperthyroidism

CAUSES

1. Diffuse toxic goitre – Graves' disease
2. Toxic nodular goitre
   i. multinodular
   ii. solitary toxic adenoma

} >90 per cent

3. Exogenous thyroid hormone
   i. overtreated myxoedema
   ii. factitious

4. Neoplastic
   i. carcinoma of thyroid
   ii. ectopic TSH-like production

5. Hashimoto's thyroiditis – transient
6. Excess TSH from a pituitary tumour

DIAGNOSIS

1. Clinical features – hands, pulse, eyes, weight loss despite good appetite
2. Serological
   i. serum T4 (thyroxine) and T3 raised
   ii. TSH concentrations are low
   iii. free thyroxine index = serum T4 × T3 resin uptake; raised
   iv. IgG antibodies directed against TSH-receptor of thyroid follicular cell

TABLE 12.1

	Graves' disease	Toxic nodular goitres
Thyroid gland	Diffuse, fleshy	Irregular nodular
Age	Younger	Older
Eye signs	Common	Infrequent
Heart signs	Not present, unless primary heart disease	Atrial fibrillation
Autoimmune associations	Common	Uncommon

Hypothyroidism

CAUSES

1. Secondary to previous ^{131}I therapy for hyperthyroidism – the most common
2. Spontaneous – chiefly in females aged 40–60 years
3. Hashimoto's thyroiditis
4. Secondary to previous surgery
5. Congenital absence occurs in 1 in 2500 to 5000 births

DIAGNOSIS

1. Clinical features – cardiac features, enlargement, failure, effusion are often missed
2. Serological
   i.   serum T4 and T3–low
   ii. serum TSH – raised; if borderline high; TRH–TSH test indicated

Causes of goitre

DEFINITION

Goitre – any enlargement of the thyroid gland. F > M especially in pre-menopausal.

1. Iodine deficiency – most common cause worldwide
2. Physiological
   i.   puberty
   ii. pregnancy

3. Graves' disease – diffusely enlarged
4. Goitrogens
   i. anti-thyroid drugs
   ii. iodine-containing medicines, lithium
5. Tumours
   i. carcinoma ⎫ rare
   ii. adenoma ⎬
6. Thyroiditis
   i. Hashimoto's
   ii. Riedel's – pressure symptoms
   iii. de Quervain's – may be painful; early transient hyperthyroidism
   iv. septic
7. Infiltrations
   i. sarcoid
   ii. tuberculosis
8. Dyshormonogenesis – a variety of conditions in which enzyme defects lead to defective thyroid hormone production

⎱ very rare

Thyroiditis

All rare

1. Acute – bacterial
2. Sub-acute (de Quervain's) – possibly Coxsackie virus B
3. Chronic
   i. Hashimoto's
   ii. Riedel's – very rare

Parathyroid glands

Actions of parathyroid hormone

1. Renal tubular reabsorption of Ca^{2+}
2. Bone turnover, especially osteoclastic reabsorption
3. Gut absorption of Ca^{2+}
4. Synthesis of $1,25(OH)_2D_3$
5. Excretion of PO_4^{3-}
6. Excretion of Na^+, K^+ and HCO_3^-

⎱ increased

The only stimulus to synthesis and release of PTH is hypocalcaemia.

Hyperparathyroidism

DEFINITION

Hypercalcaemia due to excessive production of parathyroid hormone. Serum calcium rarely greater than 3.0–3.4 mmol/ℓ (12–13.5 mg/100 ml) and serum phosphate usually not less than 0.5 mmol/ℓ (1.5 mg/100 ml).

CAUSES

1. *Primary* – caused by autonomous PTH production by
   i.   single parathyroid adenoma – >90 per cent of patients
   ii. hyperplasia or multiple adenomas – circa 8 per cent
   iii. carcinoma – circa 1 per cent

Diagnosis – Hypercalcaemia, hypophosphataemia, hypercalciuria (more than 8 mmol/24 hours; all three invariably present), raised urinary hydroxyproline (50 per cent of cases), raised serum alkaline phosphatase, raised serum PTH; renal 'stones, bones and abdominal groans'. Fatigue, muscle weakness, mental change, dehydration, conjunctival flare and corneal (at junction with sclera) calcification.

Presentation
   i. by chance on biochemical screening – the most common
   ii. acute hypercalcaemic syndrome – dehydration, confusion

2. *Secondary* – chronic PTH overproduction as a consequence of prolonged hypocalcaemia. Serum calcium either low or low normal
   i.   chronic renal failure – failure of 1,25 $(OH)_2D_3$ production
   ii. vitamin D deficiency – poor diet and lack of sunlight
   iii. steatorrhoea, following major resection of bowel

3. *Tertiary* – when the PTH production of secondary hyperparathyroidism becomes autonomous in either one or more glands
   i. chronic haemodialysis patients ⎫
   ii. postrenal transplant patients   ⎬ a minority
                                        ⎭

Hypoparathyroidism

DEFINITION

Absence of PTH, hypocalcaemia – serum calcium falls to about 1.25 mmol/ℓ (5 mg/100 ml). Raised serum phosphate concentrations and normal alkaline phosphatase activity.

CAUSES

1. Post-thyroid gland surgery
2. Neonatal – transient, self-limiting in days
3. Idiopathic – usually children, but in adults associated with pernicious anaemia identical or Addison's disease

} biochemically identical

4. Severe Mg^{2+} deficiency. Mg^{2+} required for PTH release
5. Pseudohypoparathyroidism. Rare. Failure of tissue receptors for PTH. Characteristic skeletal deformities, obesity and mental deficiency.

Tetany

DEFINITION

Excitability of peripheral nerves due either to a low serum calcium or an alkalosis which depresses ionized calcium, or both.

1. Inadequate calcium intake
    i.   prolonged poor diet
    ii. inadequate vitamin D
    iii. severe malabsorption
2. Hypoparathyroidism
3. Chronic renal failure – very infrequent
4. Alkalosis – *see* pages 62 and 67

Adrenal cortex

Diseases of the adrenal cortex

EXCESSIVE PRODUCTION

1. Glucocorticoid – Cushing's syndrome
2. Aldosterone – Conn's syndrome
3. Androgen – adrenal virilism
4. Enzyme defects – congenital adrenal hyperplasia

INSUFFICIENT PRODUCTION

1. Primary adrenal destruction – Addison's disease
2. Secondary adrenal atrophy – ACTH deficiency

Causes of Cushing's syndrome – serum cortisol concentrations increased

1. Non-ACTH dependent
   i.   corticosteroid therapy – very common (ACTH suppressed)
   ii. adenoma of adrenal cortex ⎫ 10 per cent of
   iii. carcinoma of adrenal cortex – ⎬ endogenous
        infrequent ⎭ cases
2. ACTH dependent
   i.   pituitary dependent bilateral adrenocortical hyperplasia – Cushing's disease; 70 per cent
   ii. ACTH therapy – common
   iii. ectopic ACTH production
        (a) bronchogenic carcinoma – fulminant disease, death in weeks, 5–10 per cent
        (b) bronchial carcinoid – more benign simulating Cushing's disease

CLINICAL FEATURES

1. Face – plethoric, fat, hirsute
2. Skin – acne, bruising, striae (younger patients), pigmentation
3. Trunk – obese, protuberant abdomen
4. Limbs – thin, proximal myopathy of hips and shoulder (older patients)
5. Bones – osteoporosis, kyphosis, collapsed vertebrae, growth retardation
6. Urine – polyuria, nocturia, glycosuria

7. CVS – hypertension and oedema due to salt and water retention
8. Psychological – depression, insomnia, mania or psychosis
9. Sexual function – oligomenorrhoea or amenorrhoea, impotence

DIFFERENTIAL DIAGNOSIS

1. Cushing's syndrome
2. Obesity ⎤ Circadian variation of serum cortisol con-
3. Simple hirsutism ⎬ centration maintained and urinary free
4. Alcoholism ⎦ cortisol concentration normal

Diagnostic tests

TABLE 12.2

	Pituitary dependent	Ectopic ACTH	Adenoma	Carcinoma
1. Serum cortisol, circadian rhythm	Absent	Absent	Absent	Absent
2. Plasma K^+ <3.3 and bicarbonate >30 mmol/ℓ	Unusual	Usual	Usual	Usual
3. Dextramethasone suppression of serum cortisol. Low dose (2 mg/day, 48 hours)	Absent	Absent	Absent	Absent
High dose (8 mg/day, 48 hours)	Present	Absent	Absent	Absent
4. Metyrapone blockade of cortisol synthesis (4.5 g over 24 hours)	Pronounced	Absent	Absent	Absent
5. Serum ACTH	High	Very high	Not detectable	Not detectable

OTHER TESTS

1. X-ray of pituitary
2. C T scan of adrenal glands
3. Chest X-ray – ectopic production
4. Great vein sampling for local high concentrations of ACTH

Hyperaldosteronism

1. Primary – very rare
   Conn's syndrome – adenoma of zona glomerulosa, 60 per cent. Hyperplasia; 40 per cent. Hypokalaemia <3.5 mmol/ℓ, alkalosis bicarbonate >30 mmol/ℓ, hypertension mild to accelerated

(less than 0.01 per cent of all cases of hypertension). Low peripheral venous renin activity, raised aldosterone, renal veins catheterized for aldosterone sampling.

2. Secondary

    i.   pregnancy – physiological hyperaldosteronism
    ii.   diuretic therapy
    iii. congestive heart failure
    iv. vasodilators   with oedema or
    v.   cirrhosis   hypertension
    vi. nephrotic syndrome
    vii. accelerated hypertension
    viii. liquorice   high dose
    ix. carbenoxolone
    x.   bartter's syndrome (rare)

Adrenal virilization

Overlap with glucocorticoid (Cushing's) or mineralocorticoid (Conn's) producing tumours. An uncommon condition.

CLINICAL FEATURES

1. Hypogonadism
2. Hirsuties
3. Hypertrophy of muscles
4. Enlarged clitoris

Addison's disease

DEFINITION

Inadequate production of adrenocortical hormone.

CAUSES

Chronic

1. Addison's disease – rare

    i.   autoimmune adrenal failure – F > M, adrenocortical antibodies in serum. Other organ-specific autoimmune diseases may be present. The most common cause of Addison's disease
    ii. tuberculous – much less frequent
    iii. infiltration by neoplasm or amyloid

2. Failure of ACTH production
   i.   pituitary disease
   ii. pituitary stalk disease
   iii. disease of third ventricle
   iv. after bilateral adrenalectomy for breast cancer

3. Adrenal vein thrombosis after adrenal venography

Acute
Adrenal crisis – occurs in patients having been, or being, treated with long-term corticosteroids. Precipitated by sudden withdrawal of corticosteroids, surgery, infection or bilateral adrenalectomy

Endocrine manifestations of cancer

TABLE 12.3

Ectopic hormone	Most common tumours	Clinical and biochemical features	Syndrome
ADH	Oat cell carcinoma of bronchus – 40 per cent of all cases. Pancreatic carcinoma, lymphadenoma	Hyponatraemia Drowsiness Confusion	Inappropriate antidiuresis (*see* page 68)
PTH	Squamous cell tumours Adenocarcinoma of kidney Breast and ovarian tumours	Polyuria Polydypsia Vomiting Psychosis Steroid suppressable	Non-metastatic hypercalcaemia
ACTH	Oat cell carcinoma Islet cell carcinoma of pancreas Bronchial carcinoid	Weakness Glycosuria Hypokalaemia Alkalosis	Cushing's syndrome
Renin	Lung, pancreatic or ovarian carcinoma	Hypertension $K^+ < 3.2\,mmol/\ell$	Hyperreninism

Multiple endocrine neoplasia (MEN)

Very rare. Some are familial. Some features may be absent

TYPE I

1. Islet cell pancreatic tumour – Zollinger–Ellison, producing gastrin or insulin
2. Pituitary tumour – chromophobe or eosinophil adenoma
3. Primary hyperparathyroidism – adenoma or hyperplasia
4. Adrenocortical tumour

TYPE II

1. Medullary carcinoma of thyroid
2. Hyperparathyroidism
3. Phaeochromocytoma

[handwritten annotations: "A Cush Dur" and "B Neuromas Marfanoid"]

TYPE III

Multiple mucosal and cutaneous neurofibromas

Diabetes mellitus

DEFINITION

Hyperglycaemia due to deficiency or impaired effectiveness of insulin. Chronic conditions affecting carbohydrate, lipid, protein, electrolyte and water metabolism. Two main types – insulin-dependent (IDD or type I) and non-insulin-dependent (NIDD or type II), the causes of which are quite different. Prevalence in UK is more than 1 per cent.

DIAGNOSTIC BLOOD GLUCOSE CRITERIA

TABLE 12.4

Classification	Fasting	Random	Two hours post 75 g oral glucose
Diabetes	>7.0 mmol/ℓ (>120 mg/100 ml)	>11.0 mmol/ℓ (>200 mg/100 ml)	>10 mmol/ℓ (>180 mg/100 ml)
Equivocal	all intermediate concentrations		
Normal	<6.0 mmol/ℓ (<110 mg/100 ml)	<6.0 mmol/ℓ	<6.0 mmol/ℓ

UPPER LIMITS OF NORMAL BLOOD GLUCOSE – following 75 g oral glucose; venous blood analysed by the glucose oxidase method:

Fasting	6.0 mmol/ℓ
Peak	9.0 mmol/ℓ
2 hour	6.0 mmol/ℓ

CLASSIFICATION

1. Primary (idiopathic)

    i.   IDD 'juvenile onset' – children, adolescents, young adults. Links with HLA antigens: DW3, DR4. Classical ketoacidotic diabetes

    ii. NIDD 'maturity-onset' – frequency increases with age. May present with complications of diabetes

TABLE 12.5

Comparison	Insulin-dependent	Non-insulin-dependent
Age	<40 years	Usually >40 years
Incidence	Peak 12–14 years	Peak at eighth decade
Association with HLA	Present	Absent
Association with autoimmune disease	Present	No more than chance
Ketosis	Usual	Rare
Onset	Acute or subacute	Insidious
Obesity	Uncommon	Frequent

2. Gestational – diabetic whilst pregnant, much greater risk of permanent diabetes later

3. Latent – abnormal GTT with probability of permanent diabetes in the future

4. Secondary to endocrine and metabolic disease <1 per cent of all cases

    i.   thyrotoxicosis
    ii.   Cushing's syndrome
    iii. acromegaly
    iv.   phaeochromocytoma
    v.   haemochromatosis
    vi.   glucagonoma

5. Secondary to drug therapy
   i.   glucocorticoids – common
   ii. oral contraceptives
   iii. thiazides
   iv. diazoxide

DIFFERENTIAL DIAGNOSIS OF GLYCOSURIA

1. Diabetes mellitus
2. Anxiety
3. Alimentary – lag storage
4. Renal glycosuria in pregnancy – temporarily reduced T_{mG}
5. Renal glycosuria – reduced T_{mG}
6. Caused by drugs – *see* above
7. Secondary to metabolic diseases – *see* above

TYPES OF GLUCOSE TOLERANCE TEST CURVES

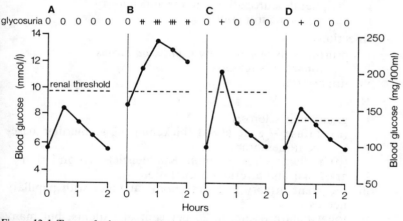

Figure 12.1 Types of tolerance test curves. A normal; B diabetic; C alimentary glycosuria (post-gastrectomy); D renal glycosuria. A similar type of curve - 'flat' or 'lag storage' – occurs as a variant of normal and in malabsorption

Complications of diabetes mellitus

STRUCTURAL

1. Cardiovascular – most common cause of death in patients >50 years

    i. atheroma of large vessels
   ii. endarteritis of small vessels
  iii. result in ischaemia of heart, brain, eyes, feet, kidneys, hypertension

2. Eye
    i. retinopathy – very common, may be asymptomatic but is the single most common cause of blindness in the middle-aged
       (a) microaneurysms
       (b) haemorrhages
       (c) exudates – hard and soft
       (d) new vessel formation around disc leading to retinitis proliferans
   ii. cataract – in adolescents and early adult life

3. Nervous system
    i. cerebral lesions secondary to atheroma – common
   ii. comas – *see* following lists and page 239
  iii. peripheral neuropathy – motor and sensory
   iv. autonomic neuropathy

4. Infections
    i. pruritus vulvae caused by *Candida albicans*
   ii. pulmonary tuberculosis
  iii. urinary tract

5. Renal
    i. glomerular sclerosis
       (a) diffuse – generalized thickening of glomerular basement membrane
       (b) nodular – less common; Kimmelstiel–Wilson lesion
   ii. arteriolar and arterial degeneration
  iii. recurrent urinary tract infections, at times with papillary necrosis
   iv. renal failure occurs in 20 per cent of patients, but many diabetics die of other complications before renal failure becomes terminal

METABOLIC

All quite frequent

1. Hypoglycaemia
2. Hyperglycaemia
    i. ketotic
   ii. non-ketotic

3. Lactic acidosis – phenformin; infrequent
4. Hypertriglyceridaemia; hypercholesterolaemia seldom occurs
5. Obesity
6. Pseudohyponatraemia – hyperglycaemia
7. Hypernatraemia ⎱ part of ketotic hyperglycaemia
8. Hypokalaemia   ⎰
9. Metabolic complications of chronic renal failure

Comas in diabetes

TABLE 12.6

Type	Plasma glucose	Ketosis	Acidosis	Dehydration	Hyperventilation
Ketoacidotic – hyperglycaemia	↑ ↑ ↑	↑ ↑ ↑	↑ ↑ ↑	Very	Prominent
Non-ketotic	↑ ↑ ↑	Nil	Nil	Very	None
Hypoglycaemic	↓ ↓	Nil	Nil	Nil	None
Lactic acidosis	↓ to ↑ ↑	Mild	↑ ↑ ↑ ↑	Some	Prominent

Differential diagnosis of a diabetic coma

TABLE 12.7

	Hyperglycaemia	Hypoglycaemia
Onset	Gradual	Sudden – excess insulin
Symptoms	Unwell, abdominal pain, vomiting	Faint, shaky, hungry, irritability
Signs	Dehydrated, small pulse, hypotension, air hunger, (acidotic respiration)	Moist, full pulse, normal breathing, dilated pupils
Urine – fresh sample required	Glycosuria, ketonuria	Normal
Blood	Hyperglycaemia acidosis	Hypoglycaemia Normal pH
Fatality	Up to 15 per cent	<1 per cent

Causes of hypoglycaemia

1. Children become hypoglycaemic more readily than adults
2. Ethanol masks symptoms so that hypoglycaemia is mistaken for intoxication

3. Exercise increases insulin absorption and promotes peripheral glucose uptake
4. Insulin requirements fall in long-term diabetics
5. The elderly do not tolerate hypoglycaemia well
6. 'Brittle' diabetics have either a tendency to hyperglycaemia or hypoglycaemia; rarely both

POST-PRANDIAL ATTACKS

1. Following gastric surgery – attacks occur 2–3 hours after meals; distinct from the 'dumping' syndrome
2. Early diabetes – late reactive hypoglycaemia
3. Idiopathic reactive hypoglycaemia

FASTING ATTACKS

1. Advanced liver disease – restricted gluconeogenesis and glycogenolysis
2. Factitious – self-administration of insulin or a sulphonylurea
3. Ethanol-induced – in fasting alcoholics
4. Hypothermia
5. Insulinoma – inappropriately raised plasma insulin
6. Large sarcomas – rare; secrete a pro-insulin peptide

Complications of diabetic pregnancy

MATERNAL

1. Hyperglycaemia and ketoacidosis
2. Hypoglycaemia
3. Pre-eclampsia
4. Pre-term labour

FETAL

1. Macrosomia
2. Neonatal – hypoglycaemia, hypocalcaemia, high PVC, jaundice
3. Respiratory distress syndrome
4. Interuterine death
5. Congenital abnormalities: clasically sacral agenesis

Gynaecomastia

DEFINITION

Enlargement of the male breast.

1. Neonatal – transient – 2 per cent
2. Puberty – 50 per cent of normal boys aged 12–15 years
3. Elderly – prevalence increases with advancing age
4. Drugs
   i.   oestrogens or androgens
   ii. spironolactone ⎱ displacement of dihydrotestosterone
   iii. cimetidine   ⎰ from its intracellular receptor
   iv. digitalis ⎫
   v.   methyldopa │
   vi. isoniazid │
   vii. phenothiazines ⎬ perhaps by unknown mechanisms
   viii.reserpine │
   ix. tricyclics │
   x.   diazepam   ⎭
   xi. cytotoxic agents – via testicular damage
5. Alcoholic cirrhosis – common
6. Hyperparathyroidism – 10–40 per cent of patients
7. Chronic renal failure – early weeks of dialysis
8. Refeeding after severe malnutrition
9. Klinefelter's syndrome – XXY, orchitis or castration
10. Pituitary failure

Amenorrhoea

No periods for more than 3 months.

PHYSIOLOGICAL

1. Pre-pubertal
2. Pregnancy
3. Athletes

PATHOLOGICAL

1. Severe generalized chronic disease
   i.   chronic renal failure ⎫
   ii. thyrotoxicosis   ⎬ common
   iii. hypothyroidism – hyperprolactinaemia ⎭

2. Pituitary disease
   i.   tumours – hyperprolactinaemia; important cause
   ii. infarction, granulomas and trauma
3. Hypothalamus
   i.   severe weight loss – 40–50 per cent of all cases
   ii. post-oral contraception
   iii. psychogenic
   iv. tumours
   v.   obesity
4. Gonadal – rare
   i.   polycystic ovarian syndrome
   ii. ovarian failure – premature menopause
   iii. testicular feminization – always primary amenorrhoea
   iv. gonadal dysgenesis – usually primary amenorrhoea

Possible endocrine emergencies

1. Diabetes mellitus
   i.   ketoacidosis
   ii. hypoglycaemia
   iii. hyperosmolar non-ketotic
   iv. lactic acidosis – phenformin; pH <7.0
2. Parathyroid glands and hyper- and hypocalcaemia
   i.   post-parathyroid surgery; hypocalcaemia
   ii. hypercalcaemia
        (a) malignant disease – the most common
        (b) primary hyperparathyroidism
        (c) overdose of vitamin D or synthetic analogues thereof
3. Thyroid gland
   i.   myxoedema coma
   ii. thyroid crisis
4. SIADH – *see* page 68
5. Diabetes insipidus – post-head injury
6. Hypopituitary coma
7. Adrenal gland
   i.   phaeochromocytoma
   ii. Addisonian crisis – usually occurs in a steroid ⎫ infrequent
        treated patient   ⎬
   iii. hypercortisolism   ⎭
        (a) ectopic ACTH
        (b) long-standing Cushing's syndrome

Chapter 13

General paediatrics

Development
TABLE 13.1

Age	Motor	Vision and fine moveme
4–6 weeks	In prone, head to one side May raise a little Large jerky movements of limbs Held sitting – round back, hands closed, thumbs in Still has placing, stepping, Moro responses	Turns to diffuse bright light Looks at dangling toy 15 cm from face Begins to watch mother's fa
3 months	Kicks legs alternately In prone, lifts head, forearms used for support Held sitting – back straight with curve in lumbar region Hands open, brought to midline Held standing, sags at knees	Visually alert Follows dangling toy Hand regard Recognizes bottle
6 months	Sits with support Takes weight on legs if held Rolls over Sits with straight back	Visually very alert Watches movements across room Reaches for toys nearby Whole hand palmar grasp
9 months	Sits for 10–15 minutes on floor Stands holding on Crawling attempted	Finger and thumb grasp Transfers objects from han hand
12 months	Can get to sitting position from lying down Crawls Pulls to stand Cruises round furniture	Precise pincer grasp, thumb and finger for small objects Watches small toy moving 3 m
18 months	Walks quite steadily Can pull wheeled toy Can stoop to pick up toys without falling	Spontaneous linear scribble Tower of 3 bricks Fixes on small toy at 3 m Hand preference emerging
2 years	Runs Climbs on furniture Stairs – 2 feet per step up and down	Tower of 6 bricks Spontaneous circular scribb Enjoys picture books Handedness developed
3 years	Rides tricycle Walks on tiptoe May stand on 1 foot for a few seconds	Tower of 9 Cuts with scissors Matches 2 or 3 primary col
4 years	Goes up and downstairs 1 foot per step Hops on one foot	Builds steps with 6 bricks Draws a man Copies cross
5 years	Skips and dances Can stand on 1 foot for 10 seconds Can hop 3 yards forward on either foot	Draws a house Copies circle, square, trian

Baby dropped back ⇒ arms extend + abduct
fingers ext + abd

Moro 0 → 5→6/12

stepping, Palmer Grasp → 3/12 } Primary or Automatic reflexes

ie -f 1 foot to ground ⇒ makes walking movements

Hearing and speech	*Social and play*
Startles to loud noise 'Stills' to bell	Sucks well Sleeps when not being fed or handled Smiles at mother by 6 weeks
Startles to loud noise, may cry Quietens to mother's voice Vocalizes May turn eyes toward sound	Responds with pleasure to friendly handling Holds rattle for few seconds if put into hand but does not look at it
Turns to mother's voice Vocalizes Responds to baby hearing tests by eye movements	Can grasp small toys Takes to mouth Sees rattle Friendly with strangers
Vocalizes deliberately to communicate	Puts hands to bottle or cup during feeding Distinguishes strangers from familiars
Knows own name and turns to it Actions show understanding of some words and simple commands	Holds arms to be dressed Puts cubes in and out of cup Waves 'bye-bye'
6–20 recognizable words Communicates wants by gesture and vocalization	Bowel control Drinks from cup. May use spoon Explores environment actively
50 words Uses own name Echolalia	Dry by day. Verbalizes toilet needs Demands adult attention No idea of sharing
Large vocabulary Immature pronunciation Many questions Likes stories	Dry by night Eats with fork and spoon Joins in play with other children
Gives acount of his doings can give name, address age	Undresses except back buttons and laces Understands taking turns, dramatic play and dressing up
Fluent speech	General behaviour more amenable Plays cooperatively with other children

Failure to thrive

Inadequate gain in weight (and length and head circumference), during infancy and pre-school years compared to predicted rate of gain from percentile charts. In spite of the many possible causes, no definite organic cause is found in about 45 per cent of cases investigated. Existing centile charts are derived from measurements of Caucasian children which must be borne in mind when monitoring the growth of Asian and African children.

1. Defective intake
   i.   feeding mismanagement
   ii. protein calorie malnutrition

2. Abnormal losses from GI tract by vomiting
   i.   hiatus hernia
   ii. pyloric stenosis
   iii. rumination
   iv. chronically raised intracranial pressure

3. Defects of absorption – of fat, carbohydrate or protein or a combination of these
   i. small intestine
      (a) anatomical
          malrotation
          reduplication
      (b) inflammatory
          bacterial overgrowth
          giardiasis
      (c) metabolic
          coeliac disease
          dissaccharide intolerance
             primary
             secondary to severe gastroenteritis
      (d) immunological – immune deficiency
      (e) sensitivity
          to cow's milk protein
          transient gluten sensitivity
      (f) miscellaneous
          tropical sprue
          protein calorie malnutrition
          protein losing enteropathy
      (g) tumours – lymphoma
   ii. pancreatic – cystic fibrosis
   iii. liver
      (a) cirrhosis
      (b) biliary atresia

4. Systemic disease other than GI tract
   i.   cardiovascular – some forms of congenital heart disease
   ii. respiratory
        (a) severe asthma
        (b) recurrent severe infections
   iii. renal
        (a) recurrent infection
        (b) renal tubular acidosis
   iv. CNS – global mental retardation
   v.   metabolic
        (a) phenylketonuria
        (b) galactosaemia
   vi. chromosomal abnormalities
   vii. low birth weight – especially if there is a history of intrauterine growth retardation
   viii. HIV infection

5. Emotional and social deprivation – in spite of apparently adequate caloric intake, children may not thrive in an uncaring environment.Increasingly recognized as a cause of failure to thrive

Weight loss

1. Insufficient food intake
   i. psychological disturbance
   ii. neglect – child abuse

2. Deficient utilization of available food
   i.   coeliac disease
   ii. cystic fibrosis
   iii. other causes of malabsorption

3. Abnormal losses from GI tract – persistent diarrhoea and vomiting of any cause

4. Infections
   i.   recurrent UTI
   ii. tuberculosis
   iii. chronic lung infection
   iv. glandular fever

5. Endocrine
   i.   diabetes mellitus
   ii. diabetes insipidus
   iii. thyrotoxicosis

6. Metabolic
    i. renal failure
    ii. hepatic failure

7. Malignant disease

Short stature

1. Genetic
    i.   racial and familial
    ii. chromosome disorders
        (a) Down's syndrome
        (b) Turner's syndrome
    iii. inherited skeletal disorders
        (a) achondroplasia
        (b) fragilitas ossium

2. Environmental
    i. intrauterine – placental insufficiency
    ii. extrauterine
        (a) malnutrition
            economic
            faulty feeding
        (b) emotional deprivation

3. Systemic disease in childhood
    i.   endocrine
        (a) hypothyroidism
        (b) growth hormone deficiency
        (c) poorly controlled diabetes mellitus
        (d) prolonged steroid therapy
    ii.   severe cyanotic congenital heart disease
    iii. malabsorption
    iv.   chronic renal disease
    v.   chronic infections
    vi.   chronic respiratory disease
        (a) severe asthma
        (b) cystic fibrosis
    vii. mental retardation – many such children with or without
          dysmorphic features are stunted in physical growth
    viii. mucopolysaccharidoses

Sexual precocity

ISOSEXUAL – FEMALE

1. Constitutional – 90 per cent
2. Intracranial tumours
3. Polyostotic fibrous dysplasia – Albright's
4. Adrenocortical tumour
5. Granulosa cell tumour
6. Teratoma

ISOSEXUAL – MALE

1. Constitutional – 10 per cent
2. Intracranial tumour
3. Adrenal hyperplasia or carcinoma
4. Testicular tumour
5. Hydrocephalus
6. Postencephalitis

HETEROSEXUAL

1. Adrenocortical tumour
2. Adrenocortical hyperplasia

Delayed puberty

FEMALE

1. Normal variation
2. Familial
3. Severe malnutrition
4. Chronic illness
5. ? Thyroid deficiency
6. Pituitary infantilism
7. Adrenogenital syndrome
8. Testicular feminization
9. Turner's syndrome

MALE

1. Normal variation
2. Familial
3. Malnutrition
4. Chronic illness

5. Pituitary infantilism
6. Cryptorchidism
7. Mumps
8. Klinefelter's syndrome
9. Male pseudohermaphroditism
10. Male Turner's syndrome

Vomiting

INFANCY

1. Posseting and ruminating
2. Feeding mismanagement
3. Infection
    i.   enteral – gastroenteritis
    ii. generalized infection
        (a) URTI
        (b) UTI
        (c) meningitis
        (d) pertussis
4. Hiatus hernia
5. Pyloric stenosis
6. Intestinal obstruction
7. Appendicitis
8. Raised intracranial pressure
9. Diabetes
10. Drugs and poisons

CHILDHOOD

1. Psychological
    i.   'periodic syndrome'
    ii. excitement
    iii. travel
2. Organic
    i.   infection
        (a) gastroenteritis
        (b) parenteral
    ii. appendicitis
    iii. intestinal obstruction
    iv. diabetes
    v.   drugs and poisons

Haematemesis

INFANCY

1. Hiatus hernia
2. Pyloric stenosis

CHILDHOOD

1. Swallowed blood from epistaxis
2. Severe vomiting from any cause
3. Hiatus hernia
4. Peptic ulceration
5. Stress ulcer – in burns
6. Oesophageal varices
7. Oesophageal foreign body
8. Blood dyscrasias
9. Drugs and poisons – especially iron

Diarrhoea

1. Infection
   i.   viral – Rotavirus is a common isolate
   ii. *E. coli*
   iii. *Shigella*
   iv. *Salmonella*
   v.   *Campylobacter*
   vi. parenteral infections – e.g. ear
2. Malabsorption
   i.   steatorrhoea
   ii. carbohydrate intolerance
   iii. cow's milk protein allergy
3. Mechanical bowel lesions
   i.   malrotation
   ii. Hirschsprung's disease
4. Inflammatory conditions of bowel
   i.   Crohn's disease
   ii. ulcerative colitis
5. Tumours – neuroblastoma
6. Tropical
   i.   amoebiasis
   ii. bilharzia

7. Miscellaenous
    i.   toddler diarrhoea
    ii. constipation with overflow
    iii. emotional 'irritable colon'
    iv. dietary indiscretion or faulty feeding
    v.   drugs and poisons

Constipation

1. Dietary
    i.   insufficient fluid intake
    ii. insufficient residue in diet
2. Bowel lesions
    i.   following anal fissure
    ii. Hirschsprung's disease
3. Emotional – parental overemphasis on potty-training
4. Hypothyroidism
5. Overdependence on laxatives
6. Hypercalcaemia
7. Lead poisoning

Blood in the stools

Classified according to level in the gut of origin of bleeding

1. Pharynx – swallowed from epistaxis
2. Oesophagus
    i.   hiatus hernia
    ii. oesophageal varices
3. Stomach
    i.   aspirin ingestion
    ii. peptic ulceration
4. Small intestine
    i.   infection – dysentery
    ii.   intussusception
    iii. Meckel's diverticulum
    iv.   reduplication cyst
    v.   polyps
    vi.   tumours
    vii. Henoch–Schönlein purpura
    viii. haemolytic uraemic syndrome
    ix.   blood dyscrasia

5. Large intestine
    i.   ulcerative colitis
    ii. constipation
6. Rectum
    i.   polyp
    ii. prolapse
    iii. foreign body
7. Anus – fissure

Recurrent abdominal pain

1. Unexplained in 95 per cent of cases. Psychological factors relevant. Periodic syndrome
2. GI tract
    i.   constipation
    ii.   peptic ulcer
    iii. food allergy
    iv.   lactose intolerance
    v.   lead poisoning
    vi.   worms
    vii. malrotation with intermittent volvulus
3. Respiratory tract – recurrent sore throats with mesenteric adenitis
4. Renal tract – urinary infection
5. CNS – temporal lobe epilepsy
6. Other – sickle cell disease

Acute abdominal pain

1. GI tract
    i.   gastroenteritis
    ii.   appendicitis
    iii. strangulated inguinal hernia ⎫
    iv.   intussusception   ⎬ especially under 1 year
    v.   volvulus
    vi.   Meckel's diverticulum
    vii. peritonitis
    viii. peptic ulcer
    ix.   gall stones – n.b. familial spherocytosis
    x.   Crohn's disease
    xi.   ulcerative colitis
    xii. infective hepatitis

2. Respiratory tract
    i. pneumonia
    ii. throat infection with mesenteric adenitis

3. Renal tract
    i. urinary infection
    ii. renal colic
    iii. Wilms' tumour – more usually presents as a mass

4. Other
    i. diabetes mellitus
    ii. Henoch–Schönlein purpura
    iii. sickle cell crisis

Headache

1. Psychological – response to school or family stresses

2. Migraine
    i. may be positive family history
    ii. may be dietary trigger factors

3. Organic illness
    i. infection
        (a) general – headache part of the malaise of systemic infection
        (b) CNS infection
            meningitis
            encephalitis
            cerebral abscess
        (c) referred pain from infection in ears, eyes, teeth or sinuses

4. Systemic disease
    i. CNS
        (a) refractive error
        (b) cerebral tumour
        (c) trauma
        (d) arteriovenous malformation
        (e) epilepsy
        (f) benign intracranial hypertension
    ii. renal – hypertension

Anaemia

1. Blood loss – usually from GI tract
2. Defective red cell production
    i.   nutritional deficiency
         (a) iron
         (b) folate
         (c) B_{12}
    ii. red cell aplasia
         (a) Fanconi's anaemia associated with congenital abnormalities
         (b) acquired secondary to drugs or toxins – *see* page 111
         (c) congenital pure RBC aplasia
    iii. marrow infiltration interfering with red cell production – leukaemia
3. Haemolysis
    i.   defects of RBC
         (a) familial spherocytosis
         (b) familial elliptocytosis
    ii. RBC enzyme deficiencies
         (a) G6PD deficiency
         (b) pyruvate kinase deficiency
    iii. defects in type or proportions of haemoglobin synthesized
         (a) sickle cell disease
         (b) thalassaemia
    iv. acquired haemolytic anaemia
         (a) autoimmune – systemic lupus erythematosus
         (b) haemolytic uraemic syndrome
         (c) drugs and poisons
4. Miscellaneous
    i.   chronic infection
    ii. renal failure
    iii. malignancy
    iv. lead poisoning

Purpura

1. Thrombocytopenic
    i.   idiopathic
    ii. post-infective – rubella
    iii. blood dyscrasias

    iv. drugs
    v. disseminated intravascular coagulation

2. Vascular
    i. Henoch–Schönlein purpura
    ii. meningococcal septicaemia
    iii. scurvy
    iv. von Willebrand's disease

3. Non-accidental injury must always be considered in cases of bruising in childhood

Lymphadenopathy

CERVICAL

1. Recurrent tonsillitis
2. Rubella
3. Infected scalp lesions

AXILLARY

1. BCG or smallpox vaccinations
2. Catscratch fever

GENERALIZED

1. Infection
    i. glandular fever
    ii. toxoplasmosis
    iii. tuberculosis
    iv. brucellosis
    v. generalized infected eczema
    vi. HIV infection

2. Malignancy
    i. leukaemia
    ii. neoplasm
    iii. reticulosis

3. Collagen disorder
    i. juvenile rheumatoid arthritis
    ii. systemic lupus erythematosus

Congenital heart disease

Classified according to type of lesion.

1. Abnormal communication between right and left sides of the heart
2. Obstructive lesions
3. Combinations of 1 and 2

May also be classified as cyanotic or acyanotic. This depends on the direction of blood flow through a shunt, right to left shunts produce cyanosis. Initially acyanotic disease may become cyanotic with reversal of direction of flow through the shunt.

1. Abnormal communications*
   i.   ventricular septal defect (VSD) (A)
   ii. VSD with pulmonary hypertension (Eisenmenger) (C)
   iii. patent ductus arteriosus   (A)
   iv. atrial septal defect
        (a) secundum (A)
        (b) primum (A)
        (c) endocardial cushion defect   (A or C)
   v.   transposition of great vessels   (C)
   vi. total anomalous pulmonary venous drainage (C) } rare
   vii. aortopulmonary window   (C)
   viii. single ventricle   (C)
   ix. truncus arteriosus   (C)

2. Obstructions*
   i.   pulmonary stenosis
        (a) valvar (A)
        (b) infundibular   (A)
   ii. aortic stenosis
        (a) valvar (A)
        (b) subvalvar (A)
        (c) supravalvar – bicuspid aortic valve (A)
   iii. coarctation of aorta (A)
   iv. left-heart syndrome (A and C)

3. Combinations*
   i.   Fallot's tetralogy (C)
   ii. mitral atresia (C)
   iii. tricuspid atresia (C)

* A = acyanotic; C = cyanotic

Respiratory disorders

The pattern of respiratory illness varies with the age of the child. Signs and symptoms relate to the level of infection in the respiratory tract, either upper or lower, although there is often some overlap.

1. Coryza
2. Tonsillitis with or without otitis media
3. Croup
4. Epiglottitis – *Haemophilus influenzae*
5. Laryngotracheobronchitis
6. Wheezy bronchitis
7. Bronchiolitis – respiratory syncytial virus is the most common isolate
8. Pneumonia
9. Pertussis
10. Asthma triggered by
    i.   infection
    ii. allergy – high IgE
    iii. stress
    iv. exercise
11. Cystic fibrosis
12. Inhaled foreign body
13. Pulmonary tuberculosis

Tendency to recurrent respiratory illnesses

1. Unexplained – usually the case
2. Asthma
3. Cystic fibrosis
4. IgA deficiency
5. Congenital heart disease with left to right shunt increasing pulmonary blood flow
6. Following pertussis
7. Retained inhaled foreign body, especially peanuts

Chromosomal disorders

Normal karyotype – 44 autosomes
　　　　　　　　　　　2 sex chromosomes – XX female
　　　　　　　　　　　　　　　　　　　 XY male

AUTOSOMAL DISORDERS

1. Trisomies in which there are three, not the usual two, of a given chromosome
    i.   Down's syndrome – trisomy 21 (mongolism)
        (a) non-disjunction – 94 per cent of cases; sporadic incidence related to increasing maternal age
        (b) mosaicism – trisomy/normal; 2.4 per cent of cases
        (c) translocation – abnormalities in parent's chromosomes likely to recur in subsequent offspring; 3.3 per cent of cases
    ii. trisomy 18 Edwards
    iii. trisomy 13 Patau
2. Deletions. Partial deletion of a chromosome may be found in a retarded child with dysmorphic features. The most commonly recognized type is 'cri du chat' syndrome – partial deletion of the short arm of chromosome 5

SEX CHROMOSOME DISORDERS

1. Turner's syndrome (gonadal dysgenesis) – karyotype 45 XO. Similar features in the male are describe as Noonan's syndrome. The karyotype however is normal male, 45 XY. It is much rarer
2. Klinefelter's syndrome – karyotype 47 XXY or XXXYY or XXYY
3. Sex chromosome mosaicism
4. Abnormalities of number – XXX or XYY

Convulsions after neonatal period

The most likely cause of convulsions varies with the age of the child. Some of the conditions listed cause recurrent convulsions. Others are associated with acute treatable illnesses and do not recur.

1. Febrile convulsions – 6 months – 5 years. Occur in 4 per cent of children
2. Idiopathic epilepsy – occurs in 0.5 per cent of schoolchildren aged 5–15 years
    i. generalized seizures
        (a) grand mal
        (b) petit mal
        (c) photosensitive
        (d) myoclonic

    ii. partial seizures
       (a) temporal lobe epilepsy
       (b) Jacksonian fits

3. Infantile spasms (hypsarrhythmia) – first year of life

4. Trauma
    i. sequelae of birth injury
    ii. head injury
       (a) accidental
       (b) non-accidental } may have subdural haematoma

5. Infections
    i.   meningitis
    ii. encephalitis
    iii. cerebral abscess
    iv. cerebral malaria

6. Metabolic
    i.   hypernatraemic dehydration
    ii. hypoglycaemia
    iii. hypocalcaemia
    iv. phenylketonuria
    v. other aminoacidurias
    vi. pyridoxine deficiency } rare

7. Cerebral tumour

8. Developmental anomalies of brain
    i. hydrocephaly
    ii. porencephaly

9. Neurodermatoses – rare
    i. neurofibromatosis
    ii. tuberous sclerosis

10. Poisons – including lead
11. Hypertension – cerebral oedema } rare

12. Sequelae of immunization

13. Episodes simulating convulsions
    i.   breath-holding attacks
    ii. hyperventilation
    iii. syncope
       (a) vasovagal attacks
       (b) paroxysmal tachycardia

Loss of consciousness

1. Overdosage of drugs and poisons
2. CNS
    i.   post-ictal
    ii. head injury
    iii. infection
         (a) meningitis
         (b) encephalitis
         (c) abscess with raised intracranial pressure
    iv. cerebrovascular accident – ruptured cerebral arteriovenous malformation
    v.   cerebral tumour

3. Metabolic
    i.   severe dehydration
    ii. diabetes
    iii. hypoglycaemia
    iv. renal failure
    v.   hepatic failure
    vi. Addison's disease

Mental retardation

Prevalence – 4 per 1000 in first year of life
              3.5 per 1000 in years 1–16

GENETICALLY DETERMINED

1. Associated with congenital abnormalities
    i. chromosomal
        (a) Down's syndrome – accounts for one-third of severe mental retardation
        (b) trisomy 13
        (c) trisomy 18   } short expectation of life
        (d) cri du chat syndrome   Del prt chr 5
        (e) Turner's syndrome   } retardation in these is
        (f) Klinefelter's syndrome } usually only mild
    ii. recognizable genetically-determined syndromes with dysmorphic features – rare
        (a) Rubinstein–Taybi syndrome
        (b) Amsterdam-type dwarfism
        (c) Prader Willi syndrome
    iii. sporadic idiopathic syndromes – dysmorphic features not fitting into a recognized pattern

2. Metabolic – some rare
    i. endocrine – congenital hypothyroidism
   ii. amino acid disorders
       (a) phenylketonuria
       (b) Hartnup disease
       (c) maple syrup urine disease
  iii. carbohydrate disorders
       (a) galactosaemia
       (b) fructose intolerance
   iv. lysomal storage disorders
       (a) lipoidoses (Tay–Sachs)
       (b) mucopolysaccharidoses
    v. leucodystrophies

3. Known CNS malformations
    i. hydrocephaly – with or without spina bifida
   ii. microcephaly
  iii. hydranencephaly
   iv. craniostenosis
    v. cortical dysplasias
       (a) tuberous sclerosis
       (b) neurofibromatosis

NON-GENETICALLY DETERMINED

Generally much more common

1. Environmental
    i. prenatal
       (a) infection
          rubella
          cytomegalovirus
          toxoplasmosis
       (b) intrauterine growth retardation
          heavy maternal smoking
          chronic maternal alcohol ingestion
       (c) maternal anticonvulsant therapy
       (d) maternal phenylketonuria
   ii. perinatal
       (a) intra and postpartum hypoxia
       (b) birth trauma
       (c) prematurity
       (d) small for gestational age with hypoglycaemia
       (e) hyperbilirubinaemia
       (f) infection – meningitis
       (g) hypernatraemia

    iii. postnatal
- (a) infection
  - bacterial meningitis
  - tuberculous meningitis
  - viral encephalitis
- (b) trauma
  - accidental
  - non-accidental
- (c) deprivation – social and emotional
- (d) hypoxia
  - cardiac arrest
  - drowning
  - status epilepticus
- (e) hypoglycaemia
- (f) hypernatraemia
- (g) hypothyroidism
- (h) hypercalcaemia

2. Isolated – mental retardation without recognizable stigmata, genetic or biochemical disorders in about 30 per cent of all cases of retardation

Degenerative brain disease

Many rare

GREY MATTER

1. Poliodystrophies
   - i.   Leigh's encephalopathy
   - ii. lipoidoses
     - Tay–Sachs'
     - Niemann–Pick's
   - iii. mucopolysaccharidoses
   - iv. Huntington's chorea

2. Polioencephalitis
   - i.   acute herpes or cytomegalovirus infection
   - ii. neurotropic virus – rabies, polio
   - iii. common specific fevers – measles, rubella
   - iv. encephalitis lethargica

WHITE MATTER

1. Leucodystrophies
    i.   metachromatic leucodystrophy
    ii. disseminated sclerosis
    iii. Schilder's disease
    iv. neuromyelitis optica – Leber's disease
2. Leucoencephalitis
    i.   subacute sclerosing leucoencephalitis with measles
    ii. para-infectious leucomyelitis – measles, rubella, varicella, post-pertussis immunization

MISCELLANEOUS

1. Organic solvent abuse
2. Lead poisoning
3. Chronic barbiturate or opiate ingestion
4. Prolonged hypoglycaemia
5. Severe uncontrolled epilepsy
6. Neurodermatoses
    i.   tuberous sclerosis
    ii. neurofibromatosis

Hypotonia

1. With weakness
    i.   benign congenital hypotonia
    ii.   hypotonic cerebral palsy
    iii. Werdnig–Hoffman's disease
    iv.   muscular dystrophy
    v.   myasthenia gravis
    vi.   Guillain–Barré syndrome
    vii. spinal cord injury
2. Without weakness
    i.   Down's syndrome
    ii.   non-specific mental retardation
    iii. severe malnutrition and malabsorption
    iv.   hypothyroidism
    v.   lipoidoses
    vi.   mucopolysaccharidoses
3. Acute disease – poliomyelitis
4. Prolonged systemic illness with immobilization

Involuntary movements

YOUNG BABIES

1. Normal
    i.   startle response
    ii. sudden jerks during sleep
    iii. jaw trembling

2. Abnormal
    i.   generalized 'jitteriness'
        (a) hypocalcaemia
        (b) hypoglycaemia
        (c) hypoxia
    ii. convulsions

OLDER CHILDREN

1. Tics
2. Hiccoughs
3. Convulsions including infantile spasms
4. Athetosis and choreoathetosis – usually in cerebral palsy
5. Chorea
6. Effect of drugs
    i.   phenothiazines
    ii. metaclopramide
7. Tremor – rare in childhood
8. Tetanus

Behaviour disorders

Classified as deviations from usually accepted patterns of normal activity appropriate to the succeeding stages of a child's development. Disorders may take a different form at different stages: feeding or sleep disturbances may present differently in the toddler and in the schoolchild.

1. Feeding
    i.   refusal
    ii. food fads
    iii. over-eating

2. Sleep
   i.   refusal to settle
   ii. wakefulness during the night
   iii. early waking
   iv. nightmares
   v.   sleepwalking

3. Elimination
   i.   enuresis
   ii. day-time wetting
   iii. constipation
   iv. encopresis

4. Relation to others – attention seeking
   i.   breath-holding attacks
   ii. temper tantrums
   iii. jealousy
   iv. aggression
   v.   undue shyness and timidity

5. Gratification habits – arise if there is lack of appropriate occupation in waking hours
   i.   head banging
   ii. rocking
   iii. hair pulling
   iv. thumb sucking } normal but may be seen as problems by
   v.   nail biting   parents and teachers
   vi. masturbation

6. Hyperactivity – child continuously active and distractable with limited attention span; related in some cases to ingestion of tartarazine dyes and other food additives; frequently associated with sleep disorders

7. Schooling
   i.   refusal – separation anxiety from mother
   ii. truancy
   iii. disruptive behaviour – may compensate for fear of failure or of teasing by peers or intellectual inability to cope with the set schoolwork

8. Drug abuse
   i.   cigarettes
   ii. organic solvents
   iii. alcohol

   iv. habit-forming drugs
- (a) cannabis
- (b) cocaine
- (c) heroin
- (d) amphetamines

Social paediatrics

NON-ACCIDENTAL INJURY (NAI)

Perinatal risk factors for families at risk
1. Age of mother at child's birth <20
2. Evidence during pregnancy of psychiatric disorder
3. Family referred to medical social worker
4. Baby admitted to SCBU
5. Midwifery staff concerned by maternal handling of baby during neonatal period
6. Mothers frequently were victims of abuse as children themselves

Factors indicating possible non-accidental cause of injury
1. Delay in seeking treatment
2. History of how injury occurred incompatible with the actual injury
3. Different story of injury told at successive interviews
4. Multiple injuries of apparently varying ages
5. Evidence of old fractures on skeletal survey
6. Characteristic still, watchful attitude of child to parents

SEXUAL ABUSE

Estimated that 10 per cent of women have had some experience in childhood

Clinical pointers
1. Vulvovaginitis
2. Wetting in previously dry child
3. Abdominal pain
4. Deterioration in school behaviour
5. Little girls said to exhibit flirtatious attention-seeking behaviour

Physical signs of vulval or anal gaping with perineal soreness which heal when the child is removed from the abusing family. Investigations include interviewing the child using anatomically correct dolls, when the child is likely eventually to indicate what physical activity took place.

PLACE OF SAFETY ORDER

Issued by a magistrate enabling the Social Services Department to remove a child from the care of his parents when there are strong grounds for suspicion that injuries suffered by the child have been inflicted non-accidentally. The 'place of safety' to which the child is removed may be a hospital in the first instance for evaluation and treatment of injuries, or a local authority children's home or more usually a foster home. The order lasts 28 days. During this time proceedings must be brought in the Juvenile Court so that the magistrates may consider the evidence and reach more long-term decisions as to the child's future.

INTERIM CARE ORDER

Extends the place of safety order a further 28 days if more time is needed to investigate circumstances of the family.

CARE ORDER

Made by the Juvenile Court when non-accidental injury is proven, placing a child in the care of the Social Services Department until the age of 18 or until the parents apply successfully for removal of the care order.

SUPERVISION ORDER

Made by the Juvenile Court when non-accidental injury is not proven but where doubt exists as to the possibility. It enables the social worker to have regular access to the child for the purpose of supporting the family and monitoring the care of the child.

A child may be taken into care voluntarily. Parents may place a child in care if they have no home or means of support. They have unlimited access and may remove the child from care at any time, should their circumstances improve.

Sudden infant death syndrome

DEFINITION

Sudden death of an infant which is unexpected by history and in whom thorough necropsy fails to demonstrate an adequate cause of death. Commonest cause of death between the ages of six months and two years. Incidence 2 per 1000 live births per annum; peak age 2–5 months.

PREDISPOSING FACTORS

1. Maternal age <20 years
2. Maternal infection in pregnancy
3. Risk increases with birth order
4. Prematurity
5. Low birthweight
6. Multiple pregnancy; triplets even greater risk than twins
7. Delivery to next pregnancy interval <3 months
8. Low socio-economic group
9. Seasonal incidence – peak in February
10. Feeding difficulty in early weeks
11. History of cyanotic episodes in early weeks
12. Admission to hospital in early weeks of life
13. Retrospectively many histories reveal minor symptoms of ill health not regarded by parents as of importance
14. Unexplained decrease in rate of weight gain

CAUSAL THEORIES

1. Historically: suffocation by 'overlaying'; cow's milk allergy
2. Central apnoea in REM sleep
3. Obstructive apnoea (hypotonia of genioglossus muscle)
4. Deficient respiratory response to rise in P_{CO_2}
5. Arrhythmia – prolonged QT interval: suggestive of possible vagal inhibition
6. Immune disorders – associated with raised serum IgE concentrations
7. Sudden overwhelming infection
8. Overheating: association with malignant hyperpyrexia
9. Inherited metabolic disorders – medium chain CoA dihydrogenase deficiency
10. NAI – 'gentle battering' implicated in some cases

Chapter 14

Neonatology

Main groups of causes of illness in neonatal period (birth – 28 days)

1. Low birth weight
2. Infection
3. Birth trauma and/or asphyxia. Clinical picture resulting from this often referred to as 'cerebral irritation'
4. Major congenital abnormalities

Problems of low birth weight

<37 weeks gestation; <2.5 kg.

1. Appropriate weight for dates
    i.   problems of temperature regulation
    ii. respiratory distress syndrome
    iii. recurrent apnoea
    iv. jaundice
    v.   bleeding tendencies especially intraventricular haemorrhage
    vi. liability to infection including necrotizing enterocolitis
    vii. hypoglycaemia
    viii. hypocalcaemia
    ix. higher incidence of congenital anomalies
    x.   late development of anaemia
    xi. complication of therapy
        (a) O_2 – retrolental fibroplasia
        (b) oxygen pulmonary damage
        (c) effects of umbilical catheterization or arterial stabs
        (d) complications of i.v. alimentation
    xii. residual neurological deficit
2. Small for dates – severity of symptoms relates to stage of gestation at which growth failure began. Effect worse if it began in second trimester rather than toward end of third
    i.   hypoglycaemia

ii. any of the preceding list if the baby is pre-term as well as small for dates
iii. subsequent small size for life if growth retardation commenced early in pregnancy

Apnoea

1. Prematurity
2. Birth asphyxia or trauma $\pm$ intraventricular haemorrhage
3. Hypoglycaemia
4. Hypocalcaemia
5. Infection
6. Continuing effects of maternal sedation
7. Hypothermia
8. Hypovolaemia
9. Anaemia

Breathlessness

1. Respiratory distress syndrome
2. Transient tachypnoea of newborn
3. Pneumonia
    i. aspiration of milk or meconium
    ii. haemolytic streptococcal infection
    iii. other
4. Pneumothorax
5. 'Cerebral irritation' – variable rate, depth and pattern of respiration
6. Congenital anomalies
    i. congenital heart disease
    ii. tracheo-oesophageal fistula
    iii. diaphragmatic hernia
    iv. congenital lobar emphysema
    v. choanal atresia
7. Acidosis

Cyanosis

1. As for breathlessness, except acidosis and transient tachypnoea of the newborn
2. Apnoea
3. Persistent fetal circulation

Convulsions

1. Intrapartum hypoxia or anoxia – cerebral oedema, ± intraventricular haemorrhage, subdural effusion
2. Infection – meningitis or septicaemia
3. Hypoglycaemia
4. Hypocalcaemia
5. Hypomagnesaemia
6. Acidosis
7. Hypernatraemia
8. Hyperbilirubinaemia
9. Pyridoxine-dependent fits and other rare metabolic disorders; galactosaemia
10. Developmental anomalies of the brain
11. Narcotic withdrawal in infant of addicted mother

Jaundice

1. Physiological
2. Jaundice of prematurity
3. Breast milk jaundice
4. Blood group incompatibility

   i.   ABO
   ii. Rhesus
   iii. other – anti-Lewis, anti-Kell, etc

5. Generalized infection – especially of urinary tract
6. Absorption of blood from large areas of bruising – e.g. cephalohaematomas
7. Hepatitis

   i.   rubella
   ii. cytomegalovirus
   iii. toxoplasmosis
   iv. α_1 antitrypsin deficiency

8. Hypothyroidism
9. G6PD deficiency
10. Galactosaemia
11. Biliary atresia

Vomiting

1. Feeding mismanagement
2. Infection

3. 'Cerebral irritation'
4. Intestinal obstruction – bile stained vomitus
5. Any severe illness of other cause including necrosing enterocolitis
6. Metabolic disorders
   i.   adrenogenital syndrome ⎫ rare
   ii. galactosaemia   ⎭

Failure to feed

1. Infection
2. Prematurity
3. 'Cerebral irritation' – poor sucking reflex
4. Jaundice
5. Heart failure
6. Breathlessness from any cause
7. Congenital anomaly – e.g. cleft palate

Vomiting blood

1. Swallowed blood from delivery or cracked nipples
2. Haemorrhagic disease of newborn
3. Trauma from nasogastric tube
4. Anticoagulants in the mother

Blood in the stools

1. Swallowed blood
2. Necrotizing enterocolitis
3. Haemorrhagic disease of newborn
4. Anticoagulants in mother
5. Local trauma from thermometer

Purpura

1. 'Traumatic asphyxia'
2. Haemorrhagic disease of newborn
3. Septicaemia
4. Intrauterine infection – rubella, toxoplasmosis, cytomegalovirus
5. Maternal ITP with antibodies

Anaemia

1. Blood loss
    i. placental bleeding
    ii. from umbilical vessels
    iii. twin to twin transfusion
    iv. iatrogenic
    v. haemorrhagic disease of newborn
2. Haemolysis
    i. Rhesus incompatibility
    ii. ABO incompatibility
    iii. severe infection
3. Defective RBC production – mainly in low birth weight infants
    i. iron deficiency
    ii. folic acid deficiency
    iii. vitamin E deficiency

Diarrhoea

1. Infection
2. Phototherapy
3. Variation in maternal diet or maternal laxatives
4. Antibiotics
5. Necrotizing enterocolitis

Transplacental viral infections

TABLE 14.1

Virus	Mother	Fetus or neonate
Rubella	May be asymptomatic	Death
		Congenital malformations
		Persistent infection
Herpes simplex	Genital infection	Disseminated neonatal
		infection
Varicella-zoster	Rash	Neonatal infection
		Occasional malformation
Coxsackie B	Asymptomatic	Neonatal infection
	Aseptic meningitis	Myocarditis
	Bornholm disease	Meningitis
Cytomegalovirus	Asymptomatic	Mental retardation
		Congenital malformations
		Persistent infection
Hepatitis B	May be a severe	Neonatal hepatitis
	hepatitis	Carrier state
HIV	May be	Death in a few
	asymptomatic	months from AIDS

Chapter 15

Neurology

Definitions of some neurological terms

Alexia. Incapacity to understand written language, usually the result of focal cortical damage or neuronal disconnection. Visual, phonemic (word sound) and semantic varieties.

Agraphia. Inability to write, from a cortical lesion; usually associated with aphasia. If an alexic patient is able to write, it appears as if he writes with his eyes closed. Such patients will write better to dictation than if copying.

Amaurosis. Loss of vision – uni- or bilateral.

Dysdiadochokinesis. Rapidly alternating movements are wild and irregular due to fragmentation of the normally smooth continuous movements.

Dysarthria. A defect of articulation resulting from neuromuscular disorders where the processes that control and co-ordinate the movements of lips, tongue and palate are involved. Stammering is not included. Anarthria is the complete inability to articulate words. The motor nuclei of the VII, IX, X, XI and XII innervate the articulatory muscles although the lesion may well be above this level.

Dysphonia. The production of incorrect vocal sounds in that the strength, tone, pitch and resonance of the voice are impaired. Articulation may be normal or abnormal. The combination of dysarthria and dysphonia is called dysarthrophonia.

Dysphasia. A linguistic disorder causing partial or complete (aphasia) disruption of expression, fluency or comprehension of speech. A lesion of the language area of the dominant cerebral hemisphere.

Dyslalia. The prolongation of immature articulation of words beyond the normal age.

Dyslexia. A disorder manifested by difficulty in learning to read despite conventional instruction, adequate intelligence and opportunity, dependent on fundamental cognitive disabilities that are frequently of constitutional origin.

Dyspraxia. The inability to perform voluntary movements in the presence of normal muscle strength.

Febrile seizure. An event in infancy or childhood (usually 3 months to 5 years of age) associated with fever but without intracranial infection or defined cause. Benign, quite separate from epilepsy which is characterized by recurrent non-febrile seizures.

Fibrillation. An EMG record of a contraction of a single muscle fibre.

Fasciculation. Brief subcutaneous contraction of bundles of muscle fibres. A sign of denervation (lower motor neuron lesion).

Locked-in syndrome. Tetraplegic and mute with preserved consciousness. Can only communicate by blinking and vertical eye movement. Results from infarction, haemorrhage or demyelination in ventral pons or medulla; pyramidal tracts to limbs and cranial nerves paralysed with tegmental sparing preserving the supranuclear pathway to the ocular motor mechanism. The patients die in weeks or months from complications of immobility rather than neocortical damage. The condition is quite different from coma, 'a state of unrousable unresponsiveness', or coma virgil, 'akinetic mutism': in both of these states the patient is motionless and mindless.

Myoclonus. Brief jerking movements of the limbs often associated with epilepsy and reflecting disease of the reticular formation or cerebellum.

Myotonia. A condition of heightened excitability of the muscle membrane. The contraction is self-perpetuating with difficulty in relaxation.

Mixed laterality. When the preferred hand and the preferred foot are not on the same side.

Tardive dyskinesia. A group of syndromes of involuntary movements arising in psychiatric patients taking neuroleptic drugs. Mostly seen in schizophrenic patients after some years of chronic neuroleptic therapy. The condition is chiefly characterized by repetitive pouting of the lips and protrusion of the tongue and is often accompanied by bizarre facial grimacing. At times widespread choreiform movements occur.

Tics. Causeless inopportune apparently purposive sudden movements. Facial and respiratory types are the most common.

Tinnitus. A sound, usually continuous, produced within the auditory system. Tinnitus can never be heard by an observer. Tinnitus is usually associated with hearing loss which may be conductive, sensorineural or a mixture of both. Secretory otitis media must be excluded in all cases.

Vertigo. An illusion of altered position of motion that may have objective manifestations.

Ocular movements

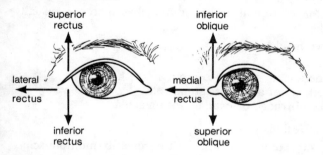

Figure 15.1 Actions of the external ocular muscles. Horizontal movement outward is abduction; inward is adduction. The recti act as elevators and depressors alone when the eye is abducted; the obliques act similarly in adduction. Nerve supply: VI – lateral rectus; IV – superior oblique; III – all the remainder including the pupil, accommodation muscles and the levator palpebrae superioris

Sudden painless visual loss

1. Central retinal artery occlusion – red spot at fovea. Segmentation of blood in vessels
2. Vitreous haemorrhage – especially retinal tear or diabetic retinitis proliferans haemorrhage
3. Central retinal venous occlusion
4. Retinal detachment
5. Acute ischaemic papillopathy – as in temporal arteritis ⎤
6. Retrobulbar neuritis ⎦ may be painful

Sudden visual deterioration in both eyes

1. Severe bilateral papilloedema of any cause – especially if haemorrhage or exudate into macula area
2. Rapidly progressive optic chiasmal compression
3. Bilateral inflammation of optic nerves – rare
4. Bilateral infarcts of occipital lobes

Visual defects due to lesions at various sites

1. Retinal lesions
   i. macular region most sensitive to alcohol, tobacco and deficiencies of B_1 and B_{12}

  ii.   choroido-retinitis
  iii. occlusion of retinal artery or branches thereof – usually embolic

2. Optic nerve head lesions
  i.   glaucoma
  ii. papilloedema – swelling of optic nerve head
    (a) oedema of adjacent retinal cells
    (b) haemorrhage or exudate into macula

3. Optic nerve lesions
  i.   acute retrobulbar neuritis – not necessarily multiple sclerosis
  ii. optic nerve compression by meningioma of olfactory groove, sphenoidal ridge or tuberculum sella – test smell, corneal reflex and III, V and VI nerves
  iii. optic nerve glioma – children and patients with neurofibromatosis
  iv. metastatic disease

4. Optic chiasmal lesions
  i.   anterior chiasmal lesions very similar lesions as in 3 ii. above
  ii. chiasmal lesions – bitemporal hemianopia with endocrine abnormalities antedating visual complaints. Causes – chromophobe adenomas (non-functioning), eosinophil adenomas (growth hormone, acromegaly), carotid syphon aneurysms, craniopharyngioma

5. Optic tract lesions – all cause homonymous hemianopias, rare
  i.   pituitary tumours
  ii. craniopharyngiomas
  iii. meningiomas

6. Optic peduncle lesions – occlusion of a thalamo-genticulate artery – rare; causes homonymous hemianopia with hemisensory loss

7. Temporal lobe lesions – tumours, abscess

8. Parietal lobe lesions – causes the rare quadrantic hemianopia; tumours, abscesses

9. Anterior visual cortex lesions – macular sparing hemianopia
  i.   migranous vascular lesions
  ii. occlusions of branch of posterior cerebral artery – rare

Visual pathways and defects thereof

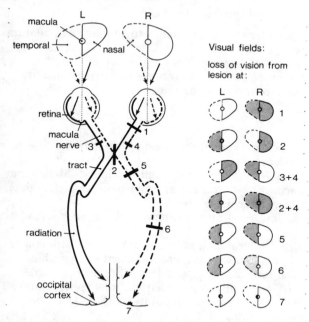

Figure 15.2 The visual pathways. Results of field testing are recorded *as seen* by the patient. *Nomenclature of lesions*: 1. Blindness of right eye; 2. Bitemporal hemianopia; 3. Binasal hemianopia; 4. Binasal hemianopia; 2 + 4. Right eye blind with temporal hemianopia of the left visual field; 5. Left homonymous hemianopia with hemianopic pupillary response; 6. Left homonymous hemianopia with normal pupillary response; 7. Left homonymous central hemiscotoma

Pupillary abnormalities

TABLE 15.1

Reaction to light	Small pupils	Large pupils
Non-reactive	Pontine bleed Opiates Pilocarpine drops Argyll Robertson (irregular)	Post-traumatic iridoplegia Mydriatic drops Holmes–Adie pupil Cerebral death Glutethamide overdose Amphetamine overdose Atropine poisoning
Reactive	Old age Horner's syndrome	Childhood Anxiety Physiological anisocoria

Horner's syndrome

Lesion in the ipsilateral sympathetic chain.

1. Pupil slightly smaller reacting normally to light accommodation
2. Some degree of ptosis
3. Enophthalmos – (sunken eyes) not easily detected
4. Conjunctiva may be bloodshot – no vasoconstrictor activity
5. Sweating over forehead may be impaired

CAUSES

1. Lesions of cervical sympathetic chain – malignant disease, surgical procedures
2. D1 root lesions – adjacent to the apical pleura. Malignancy including Pancoast's syndrome. Cervical rib (in young females), avulsion of lower brachial plexus
3. Cervical cord lesions – rare: syringomyelia, cord gliomas or ependymomas
4. Lesion of posterolateral area of brainstem – often with contra-lateral loss of pain and temperature (adjacent to spinothalamic tract). Vascular lesions, multiple sclerosis, pontine gliomas
5. Hemisphere lesions – massive infarction, hemi-spherectomy
6. Miscellaneous – congenital, migraine-associated, cavernous sinus and orbital lesions

Causes of papilloedema

1. Raised intracranial pressure due to cerebral tumours
2. Accelerated phase hypertension
3. Due to cerebral oedema
    i.   post-head injury
    ii. post-cerebral anoxia
    iii. benign intracranial hypertension
    iv. steroid withdrawal

4. Due to abnormalities of circulation – impaired venous drainage in part
    i.   central retinal vein thrombosis
    ii. SVC obstruction
    iii. polycythaemia rubra vera
    iv. multiple myeloma and macroglobulinaemia
    v.   diabetes mellitus and hyperlipidaemias
    vi. lateral sinus and jugular vein thrombosis
    vii. orbital tumours

5. Due to raised CSF protein or altered blood
   i. post-subarachnoid haemorrhage
   ii. post-meningitis
   iii. Guillain–Barré syndrome
   iv. spinal cord tumours
6. Metabolic disorders
   i. hypercapnia
   ii. diabetes mellitus
   iii. malignant thyrotoxic exophthalmos

Vertigo

DEFINITION

A hallucination of movement with rotation, swaying or falling. It is immaterial whether the patient feels the environment or he is on the move.

MAJOR CAUSES

1. Benign positional vertigo – chiefly in middle age, usually when getting up or lying down
2. Vestibular neuronitis – common, tends to occur in epidemics, may last weeks
3. Migraine – nausea, headache and vertigo
4. Brain stem ischaemia – commonest symptom of hind brain ischaemia
5. Drugs – including ethanol, sedatives, anticonvulsants and gentamicin
6. Multiple sclerosis – vertigo usually with diplopia or facial numbness, dysarthria, or weakness and ataxia
7. Menière's disease – rare, elderly, sudden, auditory symptoms essential
8. Temporal lobe epilepsy – occasional

Nystagmus

DEFINITION

Weakness in maintaining the conjugate deviation of the eyes or an imbalance in the postural control of eye movements. The slow drift component is pathological, not the fast flick.

CAUSES

1. Miscellaneous
   i.   sedatives, alcohol, anticonvulsants
   ii. transiently after recovery of consciousness after head injury
   iii. Wernicke's encephalopathy
2. Vestibular disease – any lesion affecting the semi-circular canals, VIII nerve and vestibular nuclei. The quick component is away from the side of the lesion
   i.   acute labyrinthitis – viral
   ii. vascular lesions – usually unilateral
   iii. tumours including the acoustic nerve tumour – rare
3. Cerebellar lesions
   i.   metastatic malignant disease – lung, breast and bowel
   ii. degenerative disease associated with cancer – rare
   iii. primary tumours – especially in children
4. Congenital – often familial, no fast and slow phases
5. Positional – vertigo upon lying, sitting up or turning over

Cerebral hemisphere disease

There are three basic types of lesion

1. Vascular lesions – occlusions, haemorrhage, emboli, subdural and extradural clots
2. Infiltrative or compressive tumours – primary and secondary
3. Diffuse neuronal dysfunction – metabolic and degenerative disease

Vascular lesions tend to occur in specific vascular territories; neoplastic lesions tend to occur in lobes of the brain.

FRONTAL LOBE LESIONS

TABLE 15.2

Symptoms	·Signs
Personality change	Intellectual impairment
Epilepsy	Memory defect
Loss of micturition control	Grasp reflexes
Weakness of legs – parasagittal	Motor defect – both legs or hemiplegia
Blind eye – sub-frontal lesion	Loss of smell in one nostril
	Optic atrophy and blind eye

PARIETAL LOBE LESIONS

TABLE 15.3

Symptoms	Signs
Sensory seizures	Cortical sensory loss
Dysphasia (dominant hemisphere)	Sensory inattention
Dressing apraxia ⎱ (non-dominant hemisphere)	Attention hemianopia
Geographical confusion ⎰	Dysplasia or dyspraxia

OCCIPITAL LOBE LESIONS

TABLE 15.4

Symptoms	Signs
Seizures with flashing light aura	Homonymous field defects
Visual field defects	Dyslexia or alexia
Dyslexia ⎱ area involvement	
Visual agnosia ⎰	

TEMPORAL LOBE LESIONS

TABLE 15.5

Symptoms	Signs
Epilepsy	Upper quadrantic hemianopia
Personality change	Weakness of face muscles
Memory disturbance	Hemiparesis – late

Common sites of extracranial atheroma

1. Bifurcation of common carotid in neck ⎱
2. Siphon of internal carotid artery ⎸ produce transient
3. Origin of internal carotid ⎸ hemiparetic
4. Origin of left common carotid ⎰ ischaemic attacks
5. Origin of vertebral artery – lead to brain stem ischaemic attacks
6. Proximal part of sub-clavian artery – lead to 'subclavian steal'; rare

The branches of these arteries anastomose over the cortex; clinically important impairment in any one is often critical in determining the final outcome of a major vessel occlusion.

Intracerebral vascular lesions

ANTERIOR CEREBRAL ARTERY OCCLUSIONS

Rare, urinary incontinence, flaccid weakness of leg with extensor plantar response and brisk reflexes. Touch, perception and joint position lost.

MIDDLE CEREBRAL ARTERY OCCLUSIONS

1. Main trunk – massive infarction of bulk of hemisphere. Coma with flaccid weakness of face and arm, hemianaesthesia and hemianopia; recovery remote, death frequent
2. Perforating artery (a lenticulostriate) – internal capsule area. Commonly tends to have a good prognosis. Flaccid hemiparesis, mild UMN VII. Flexor muscles of arm and extensor groups in leg become strong. Extensor plantar, sensory and field defects infrequent – supplied by posterior cerebellar artery
3. Terminal branch occlusions
   i. dominant hemisphere – damage to motor areas of face, arm and Broca's speech area. Comprehension unimpaired. Frustration. If the posterior parietal artery is occluded complete aphasia with loss of comprehension occurs but the patient may phonate single irrelevant words
   ii. non-dominant hemisphere – similar features but dysphasia is replaced by dyspraxia

POSTERIOR CEREBRAL ARTERY OCCLUSIONS

1. Main vessel – variable because of anastomoses with the middle cerebral arteries
2. Perforating artery – hemianaesthesia with loss of all modalities, complete hemianopia. The numbness may be replaced by severe painful sensations (Déjérine–Roussy syndrome). If the upper brain stem is involved hemiballismus occurs – very rare

Cardiac sources of embolism to the brain

Left atrium
1. Thrombus
2. Myxoma – very rare

Mitral valve
1. Bacterial endocarditis
2. Rheumatic endocarditis
3. Marantic endocarditis
4. Prosthesis

Left ventricular mural thrombosis
1. Myocardial infarction
2. Cardiomyopathy

Aortic valve
1. Bacterial endocarditis
2. Rheumatic endocarditis
3. Marantic endocarditis
4. Sclerosis with calcification
5. Prosthesis
6. Syphilis

Congenital heart disorders

Causes of a stroke in a young person

1. Migraine
2. Embolic
3. Thrombotic
4. Arteritis
5. Unknown – tend to do well
6. Syphilis

Subarachnoid haemorrhage (SAH)

CAUSES

1. Aneurysms of circle of Willis and its major branches–coma
2. Angiomas – arterial, capillary or cavernous; less common
3. Cranial trauma

FEATURES

1. Premonitory headache for a few days, but usually acute with severe headache, acute nausea and vomiting
2. Neck stiffness – may be absent
3. Variable level of consciousness
4. Glycosuria and transient arrhythmias – unexplained

SITES OF ANEURYSMS

1. Internal carotid circulation – 40 per cent
2. Anterior cerebral artery – 35 per cent
3. Middle cerebral artery – 20 per cent
4. Posterior circulation – 5 per cent

PROGNOSIS

Twenty-five per cent of patients die within 24 hours. A further 25 per cent die in the first month due to recurrent bleeding. The remaining 50 per cent survive with a risk of rebleeding of 2 per cent per year.

Common intracranial tumours

Ninety-five per cent of intracranial tumours can be detected by CT scanning. The CNS is the second most common site of primary neoplasms in children, in whom 70 per cent occur below the tentorium cerebelli; in adults most intracranial tumours develop above the tentorium.

TABLE 15.6

Type	Percentage incidence
Glioma	45
Meningioma	20
Pituitary adenoma	10
Acoustic schwannoma	10
Congenital	5
Vascular	5
Metastatic	10–15

Dementia

DEFINITION

A decline of intellect, personality and behaviour with disturbance of memory, orientation and capacity for conceptual thought. Called pre-senile if diagnosed before 65 years and senile beyond 65. Affects 10 per cent of the population over 65 years; half require institutional care.

CAUSES

T = treatable or possibly treatable

Intracranial
1. Alzheimer's – the majority; degeneration of ganglion cells, senile plaques, intraneuronal fibrillary tangles

2. Sub-dural – fairly common, occurs in elderly and alcoholics   T
3. Tumours, primary and secondary   T
4. Cerebrovascular disease
5. Normal pressure hydrocephalus
6. Cerebral syphilis   T
7. Brain abscess T
8. Huntington's chorea – very rare, autosomal dominant

Extracranial
1. Endocrine or metabolic
   i.   myxoedema   T
   ii. hypo- or hypercalcaemia   T
   iii. hepatic encephalopathy   T
   iv. hyponatraemia   T
   v.   dialysis dementia
   vi. carcinomatous neuropathy
2. Drugs
   i.   barbiturates or bromides   T
   ii. alcohol   T
   iii. organic poisons, solvents (glue sniffing) T
3. Vitamin deficiency
   i. B_{12} or folate   T
   ii. thiamine – alcoholics   T

Movement disorders
1. Tremor – constant rhythm, steady but variable amplitude
   i.   at rest
        (a) anxiety, alcohol
        (b) thyrotoxicosis
        (c) Parkinsonism – including drug-induced
        (d) benign essential
        (e) Wilson's disease – rare
   ii. intention tremor
        (a) multiple sclerosis
        (b) stroke
        (c) severe Parkinsonism
        (d) severe essential tremor
        (e) cerebellar disease
2. Chorea – sudden rapid involuntary, purposeless jerks
   i.   Sydenham's – rare, rheumatic fever
   ii. as a complication of SLE or thyrotoxicosis
   iii. Huntington's – rare, dominant, associated with dementia

3. Hemiballismus–wild flinging movements, especially of arm; rare
   i.   vascular damage of subthalamic nucleus
   ii. upper brain stem lesion
4. Athetosis – slow, writhing sinuous movements of arms and legs
   i.   cerebral palsy – common
   ii. post-cerebral anoxia
   iii. Wilson's disease – rare
5. Dystonias – slow prolonged contractions of trunk muscles
   i.   post-hypoxic
   ii. phenothiazines and levodopa
   iii. post-hemiplegia
6. Tics – repetitive, stereotyped brief contractions usually of face or shoulders. May be temporarily suppressed by will-power
7. Myoclonus – irregular or rhythmical muscle jerk originating in the CNS
   i.   physiological
   ii. metabolic – renal, hepatic or respiratory failure
   iii. essential (familial)
   iv. in idiopathic generalized epilepsy

Peripheral neuropathy

A disorder of peripheral nerves, sensory, motor or mixed, usually symmetrical which tends to affect distal parts of limbs. Tendon jerks are depressed or absent. Many cases are idiopathic. Diabetes, alcohol, vitamin deficiencies, drugs and malignancy are the five most common causes. There are two types of pathological processes which affect peripheral nerves

Axonal degeneration (A), the most common – the metabolism of the neuron is affected, resulting in dying-back of the distal portion of the axon
Segmental demyelination (M) results from disease of the Schwann cell or from a direct attack on the myelin with destruction of the sheath leaving the axon intact

1. Metabolic causes
   i.   diabetes mellitus – loss of vibration sense; pain – A or M
   ii. uraemia – infrequent; inadequate dialysis – A
   iii. amyloid – rare – A
   iv. myxoedema – rare – A
   v.   porphyria – very rare – A

2. Deficiency diseases – A
   i.   thiamine ⎫
   ii. nicotinic acid ⎬ chiefly in alcoholics
        ⎭
   iii. vitamin B_{12} – SACD
   iv. vitamin B_6 – isoniazid therapy
3. Drugs and chemicals – A
   i.   vincristine and vinblastine
   ii.   perhexilene maleate
   iii. isoniazid – slow acetylators
   iv.   metronidazole – for more than 2 months therapy
   v.   nitrofurantoin – in renal failure
   vi.   cisplatin
   vii. many organic chemicals – e.g. triorthocresyl phosphate
   viii. lead – rare; motor-wrist and foot drop
   ix.   Spanish cooking oil illness
4. Neoplastic causes – A
   i.   bronchial carcinoma ⎫ non-metastatic neuropathy
   ii. malignant lymphomas ⎬ is very rare
5. Infectious causes
   i.   Guillain-Barré syndrome – CSF protein raised to 30 to 100.0 g/ℓ – M
   ii. leprosy – depigmented anaesthetic areas; most common world wide cause of neuropathy
        (a) tuberculoid – A
        (b) lepromatous – M
6. Inherited causes – rare – M
   i.   peroneal muscular atrophy – Charcot–Marie–Tooth; primarily motor
   ii. hypertrophic interstitial – very rare, ulnar and lateral popliteal nerves especially easily palpable

Compression (entrapment) neuropathies

1. Carpal tunnel syndrome (median nerve) – pain, paraesthesiae, weakness and wasting of thenar eminence except the adductor pollicis
2. Ulnar neuropathy – usually following fracture dislocation of medial epicondyle of humerus
3. Meralgia paraesthetica – lateral cutaneous nerve of thigh; obesity, pregnancy
4. Tarsal tunnel syndrome (posterior tibial nerve)

Causes of subacute nerve compression

1. Prolonged recumbency – sleep, anaesthesia, coma (alcohol)
2. Haematoma – anticoagulants, haemophilia
3. Polyneuropathy – diabetes, alcoholism
4. Tourniquet palsy

Tinnitus

1. Degeneration of the organ of Corti – the most common
2. Wax in meatus
3. Otosclerosis ⎫
4. Menière's disease ⎬ often with distortion of hearing
5. Hearing loss induced by industrial noise
6. Ototoxicity from aminoglycosides
7. Temporal lobe lesions – occasionally

Spinal cord conditions

INTRINSIC (INTRAMEDULLARY) DISEASES

1. Multiple sclerosis
2. Vascular disease – especially atheroma of anterior spinal artery leading to central medullary ischaemia
3. Motor neuron disease – rare; no sensory deficit
4. Radiation myelopathy
5. Cord tumours – gliomas, ependymomas
6. Friedreich's ataxia – recessive inheritance
7. Sub-acute combined degeneration – lack of B_{12}, usually post-gastric surgery
8. Syringomyelia – rare; cavitation of central cord including hindbrain
9. Tabes dorsalis – rare

INTRASPINAL EXTRAMEDULLARY DISEASE

Tumours

1. Secondary deposits
2. Meningioma – mid-dorsal region
3. Neurofibroma – cord lesion, more common than cauda equina

Inflammatory

1. Tuberculous meningitis
2. Arachnoiditis – post-meningitis and ? contrast media

SKELETAL DISEASES

1. Cervical spondylosis – of no importance unless symptomatic
2. Secondary deposits ⎱ pain common, variable degrees of cord
3. Myeloma ⎰ compression
4. Osteoporotic vertebral collapse
5. Thoracic disc – uncommon, usually between T4 and T8
6. Lumbar spondylosis – sciatic symptoms
7. Alanto-axial dislocation – in rheumatic arthritis
8. Pott's disease – TB

Coma

DEFINITION

Failure to open the eyes either spontaneously or in response to noise, failure to obey commands, failure to move limbs in response to painful stimuli; all for at least six hours. Not all the conditions below may fit these criteria. Mortality and morbidity of non-traumatic cases of brain injury coma is very high.

1. Drugs
   i.   analgesics
   ii. anti-depressants
   iii. hypnotics
   iv. alcohol

   often taken in combination; pupillary reflexes equal, respiration depressed or Cheyne–Stokes, hypotonic limbs; *symmetrical* signs, reticular formation depression

2. Head injury
   i.   direct brain damage
   ii. sub-dural haematoma

   may well have *asymmetrical* signs due to unilateral hemisphere lesions

3. Vascular
   i.   cerebral haemorrhage
   ii. thrombosis
   iii. embolism
   iv. subarachnoid haemorrhage
   v.   hypertensive encephalopathy
   vi. major vessel occlusion

   all may well have *lateralizing* signs

4. Metabolic – all have *symmetrical* signs

   i.   hypo- (sudden) or hyper- (gradual) glycaemia – both common, easily differentiated

ii. respiratory failure – hypercapnia ⎫
iii. li\er failure – hypokalaemia and opiates ⎪ straight-
     potentiate the coma   ⎬ forward to
iv. cardiac failure – terminal   ⎪ distinguish
v.   renal failure – infrequent   ⎭
vi. hypothermia – solitary, elderly in winter

5. Epilepsy – a period of altered consciousness follows grand mal epilepsy
6. Acute infections – bacterial, AAFB, encephalitis; raised intercranial pressure
7. Space occupying lesions – neoplasm, meningioma, haematoma, abscess; with intracranial shifts and possible herniation of the tentorium cerebelli. Signs of hemiparesis, papilloedema with or without III nerve signs are very likely to be present
8. Cerebral anoxia – diffuse cortical depression, seizures with relative preservation of brain stem reflexes

Diagnosis of brain death

1. Patient is deeply comatose. Depressant drugs, hypothermia, metabolic or endocrine causes have to be excluded
2. Ventilation has to be maintained because of absence of spontaneous respiration. Muscle relaxant drugs must be excluded as a cause
3. Clear explanation of irremediable structural brain damage must be available, with loss of brain stem function

DIAGNOSTIC TESTS

Brain stem reflexes absent as shown by

1. Fixed unresponsive pupils, not necessarily widely dilated
2. Absent corneal, eyelash and blink reflexes
3. Vestibulo-ocular reflexes absent – Doll's head manoeuvre negative; caloric stimulation negative. No jaw jerk
4. No pharyngeal (gag) or laryngeal (cough) reflex
5. Cessation of respiration – diagnosed by switching off the respirator for 5 minutes while oxygen is supplied via a tracheal catheter at 6ℓ/minute. The Pa_{CO_2} should reach $50\,mmHg$ $(6.65\,kPa)$ at the end of this test, and no respiratory movements should occur

Note

1. The above tests are usually repeated at an interval of 12 or 24 hours
2. Spinal reflexes may be present; they are independent of brain stem death
3. EEG confirmation is unnecessary

Diseases of muscle: myopathies

Rare

INHERITED (GENETIC)

1. Muscular dystrophies
2. Myotonic
3. Metabolic
4. Periodic paralysis

ACQUIRED

1. Toxic
2. Inflammatory
3. Endocrine
4. Subnutrition
5. Overactive mitochondria

GENETIC

Muscular dystrophies

1. Duchenne – severe, early, most common; X-linked recessive
2. Becker – milder, presents later;   X-linked
3. Limb girdle – less common;   autosomal recessive
4. Facio-scapulo-humeral – long course;   autosomal dominant
5. Distal myopathy – late onset, very rare;   autosomal dominant

Myotonic disorders

Myotonia congenita (myotonic muscular dystropy); autosomal dominant – adults, difficulty in relaxing grip, frontal baldness, ptosis, facial weakness, testicular atrophy, conduction defects, hypoventilation, intellectual deterioration   cataract

Metabolic myopathies – the best examples include   – all A Recessive

1. Abnormalities of glycogen storage (Pompe's disease)
2. Debranching enzyme disease
3. Myophosphorylase deficiencies (McArdle's syndrome)

Familial periodic paralysis

Hypo- hyper- or normokalaemic types – all autosomal dominant

TOXIC MYOPATHIES

1. Alcohol
2. Drugs
   i.   corticosteroids – triamcinolone especially
   ii. heroin, amphetamine, clofibrate, chloroquine, vincristine, cimetidine
   iii. secondary to chronic hypokalaemia: diuretics, purgative abuse, carbonoxolane liquorice

INFLAMMATORY MYOPATHIES

1. Polymyositis – dermatomyositis; about 10 per cent are neoplasm associated
2. Secondary to
   i.   rheumatoid arthritis
   ii. systemic lupus erythematosus
   iii. systemic sclerosis
   iv. Sjögren's syndrome

3. Acute viral myositis – childhood and adolescence

Polymyalgia rheumatica – relatively common in older age groups

ENDOCRINE MYOPATHIES

1. Hyperthyroidism – proximal, fairly common
2. Hypothyroidism – occasionally mild proximal
3. Osteomalacia
4. Cushing's, Conn's, acromegaly

SUBNUTRITION

Kwashiorkor

OVERACTIVE MITOCHONDRIA

Malignant hyperpyrexia post-anaesthesia

Metabolic bone disease

1. Anticonvulsant therapy
2. Malabsorption syndromes
3. Chronic renal failure
4. Vitamin D deficiency
5. Distal renal tubular diseases

all result from very chronic states, usually all have osteomalacia, waddling gait due to painful pelvic musculature

'Queer turns'

CHILDREN

1. Petit mal and other epilepsy
2. Hypoglycaemia
3. Breath-holding attacks

ADOLESCENTS AND ADULTS

1. Vasovagal attacks – the most common
2. Hypoglycaemia
3. Dysrhythmias
4. Dumping syndrome
5. Hypocalcaemia – following hyperventilation
6. Hysteria
7. Phaeochromocytoma – rare

ELDERLY PATIENTS

1. Cerebral events related to atheroma or embolism
2. Dysrhythmias
3. Micturition syncope
4. Cough syncope

CSF findings in bacterial meningitis

1. Turbid
2. Pleocytosis – up to $1.0 \times 10^9/\ell$ more than 80 per cent polymorphs
3. Protein raised up to $1\,g/\ell$
4. CSF glucose $<2.1\,mmol/\ell$; 40 per cent below blood glucose sampled at the same time

Causes of raised CSF protein concentrations

Moderately

1. Acute bacterial meningitis
2. Multiple sclerosis
3. Early Guillain–Barré syndrome
4. Carcinomatous meningitis
5. Syphilis

Substantially

1. Froin's syndrome
2. Late Guillain–Barré syndrome
3. Acoustic neuroma

Facial pain

History important in making the diagnosis

1. Diseases of teeth, sinuses, ears or throat
2. Temporal arteritis – needs immediate prednisolone
3. Post-herpetic neuralgia
4. Facial migraine syndromes
5. Trigeminal neuralgia – rare
6. Temporo-mandibular arthritis
7. Traction headache
8. Glaucoma
9. Atypical facial pain – psychiatric

Dermatomes of head and neck

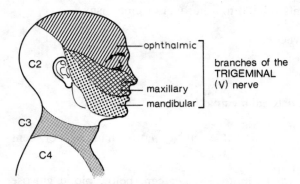

Figure 15.3 Cutaneous areas supplied by sensory roots

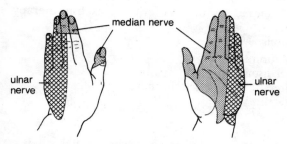

Figure 15.4 Patterns of cutaneous sensory loss after section of ulnar or median nerves in the arm. There is variation in territory supplied from person to person

Signs of peripheral nerve injury in the arm

MEDIAN NERVE DAMAGE

1. Wasting of front of forearm ⎱
2. Pointing of index finger ⎰ in forearm
3. Wasting of radial half of hand
4. Paralysis of opponens pollicis ⎱
5. Loss of sensation as above ⎰ at wrist

RADIAL NERVE IN ARM — wrist drop

ULNAR NERVE AT WRIST

1. Claw hand
2. Wasting of intrinsic muscles
3. Paralysis of abductor digiti minimi
4. Paralysis of flexor digiti minimi
5. Loss of sensation as above

ULNAR AND MEDIAN NERVES AT WRIST

1. Claw hand
2. Radial flattening
3. Sensation loss

Transient ischaemic attacks

Acute, transient episodes of focal neurological or retinal dysfunction lasting less than 24 hours presumed to be thromboembolic in origin.

1. Atheromatous plaques in neck arteries – aspirin therapy, especially in men
2. Myocardial lesions
   - i.   atrial fibrillation ⎫
   - ii. mitral valve disease ⎬ warfarin therapy
   - iii. recent infarct   ⎬
   - iv. cardiomyopathy   ⎬
   - v.   fibrin emboli   ⎭

Intracerebral abscess

Most commonly found at the junction of the cortex and sub-cortical region. Has a high mortality and morbidity; there is a high probability of epilepsy in the survivors. Streptococci and pneumococci are the commonest organisms recovered. Staphylococci are found in metastatic cases and in cases of local trauma.

CAUSAL FACTORS

1. Chronic ear infections – in 50 per cent
2. Chronic sinus infections – in 10 per cent
3. Bronchiectasis – in 20 per cent
4. Congenital heart disease with R to L shunts – in 10 per cent
5. Distant osteomyelitis   ⎫ occasionally
6. Subacute bacterial endocarditis ⎭
7. Unknown origin – in up to 20 per cent of patients

Clinical states where a sub-dural haematoma may be missed

1. In association with a head injury when improvement is slower than expected
2. People in whom head injuries often go unrecorded
   - i.   chronic alcoholics
   - ii. chronic epileptics
   - iii. boxers
3. Confused elderly patients thought to have had strokes
4. Acutely ill and chronically ill infants without external bruising
5. Post-head injury epilepsy
6. Abnormalities of blood coagulation

Lower motor neuron lesions of the VII cranial nerve

1. Idiopathic – two-thirds of cases – Bell's palsy. All patients with partial palsy recover as do three-quarters with complete palsy. Bad prognostic signs

    i.   paralysis of stapedius muscle
    ii. severe taste impairment
    iii. reduced lacrimation

2. Intracranial

    i.   metastatic malignant disease
    ii. tumours of cerebropontine angle
    iii. multiple sclerosis
    iv. infarction of brain stem

3. Temporal bone

    i.   fractures*
    ii. surgical procedures*
    iii. otitis media*
    iv. acoustic neuroma
    v.   Ramsay Hunt syndrome – herpes zoster*
    vi. carcinoma of middle ear

4. Extracranial

    i.   tumours of parotid gland
    ii. trauma*
    iii. sarcoid
    iv. mononucleosis
    v.   Bell's palsy*

Principal root values of arms and legs

TABLE 15.7

Root	Muscle	
C5/6	Biceps	
C6	Brachioradialis	
C7	Triceps	
C8	Finger flexors	tendon reflexes
L3/4	Quadriceps	
S1/2	Gastrocnemius and soleus	
T8–12	Anterior abdominal	
L1/2	Cremasteric	
S1	Plantar	superficial reflexes
S3/4	Anal	

* Most common causes

Headache

Few patients with headaches have serious disease. History most important in making the diagnosis.

1. Tension headache – common; 'scalp too tight'; no signs
2. Migraine – recurrent attacks of headache varying in frequency, duration and intensity. Tends to be unilateral at onset and proceeded by sensory, motor or mood disturbance. Nausea and vomiting common. Often familial
   i.   classical – hemicrania
   ii. common migraine – no aura; common
   iii. hemiplegic migraine – rare; hemiparetic prodrome
   iv. ophthalmoplegic migraine – usually III nerve affected
3. Migrainous neuralgia – strongly lateralized, clusters of attacks, lacrimation
4. Traction – intercranial arterial displacement and dural distortion
   i.   intracranial bleeding
   ii. tumours
   iii. post-lumbar puncture
5. Inflammation – meningitis

Wernicke's encephalopathy (mid-brain encephalopathy)

1. Nystagmus
2. Extra-ocular nerve palsies } respond to thiamine therapy
3. Dysarthria
4. Memory deficit including confabulation – the latter is striking but not diagnostic. It is referred to as Korsakoff's syndrome
5. Ataxia
6. Gaze palsies

Disorders of potency

Erection requires an intact parasympathetic reflex arc at S2/3. Ejaculation is controlled via the sympathetic L1 root.

CAUSES OF LOSS OF POTENCY

1. Psychic – anxiety, depression, psychosis

2. Autonomic nerve lesions
   i.   diabetes mellitus
   ii. ganglion blocking drugs and other hypotensive drugs functioning at adrenergic nerve endings
   iii. crush fractures of L1
   iv. chronic polyneuropathy of any cause
   v.   Shy–Drager syndrome – rare

3. Spinal cord lesions
   i.   compression
   ii. transection
   iii. MS
   iv. posterior column disorders

4. Endocrine disorders – potency is affected in many endocrine diseases

5. Cauda equina lesions
   i.   compression
   ii. transection
   iii. tumours

Chapter 16

Immunology

Immune responses are distinguished from non-specific host defence by

1. Specificity of the reaction – both antibody and cellular
2. Memory, such that a second exposure to an antigen causes both a more rapid and vigorous immune response

Effects of immune events are

1. Antibody (humoral) dependent; from B-cells
2. Cell-mediated response (CMI); from T-cells

Both B- and T-cells react with each other and antigen presenting cells.

Mediators of immunity

TABLE 16.1

Cellular		Humoral
Polymorphs		Immunoglobulins – from B-cells
Macrophages	} antigen presenta-	Complement
Dendritic cells	} tion to T-cells	Lymphokines – from T-cells
Mast cells		
Lymphocytes		
i. T-cells – high binding affinity for antigen. About 80 per cent of circulating lymphocytes. Subsetted into T-helper/inducer and T-cytotoxic/suppressor cells		
ii. B-cells – production of specific antibody molecules (plasma cells)		
iii. K-cells – lyse antibody-coated cells by attaching to the Fc end of the antibody molecule. Cytotoxic T-cells		

Lymphokines and their properties

Soluble substances liberated from activated lymphocytes the majority of which are T-cells or monocytes.

1. Macrophage inhibition and activation factors – reduces macrophage motility and increases phagocytosis
2. Neutrophil chemotactic factors – attraction of polymorphs
3. Transfer factor – activation of other lymphocytes
4. Cell growth inhibitors – prevents cell proliferation
5. Interferon γ – blocks viral reproduction and increases HLA antigen expression
6. Lymphocytotoxin – cell death
7. Interleukin-1 (IL-1) – IL2 release and B-cell maturation
8. Interleukin-2 (IL-2) – stimulates T-cells, specific receptor

T- and B-lymphocytes

TABLE 16.2

T-cells	B-cells
Cell mediated immunity – against intercellular organisms and transplanted organs	Humoral immunity – against encapsulated pyogenic bacteria
Principally circulating – 80 per cent of normal lymphocytes	Majority fixed and immobile – 20 per cent circulate
Found in perifollicular areas of deep cortex of lymph nodes	Present in germinal centre of lymph nodes
Most are long lived 'memory' cells	2–3 day life span – plasma cells
T specific surface membrane antigens	Surface immunoglobulins
A series of different subtypes identified serologically	Have membrane receptors for Fc fragment of IgG, immune complexes and C3
Two main types: effector T-cells which mediate cytotoxicity and DH; regulator T-cells which amplify or suppress immune response	Precursors of antibody secreting plasma cells

252   Immunology

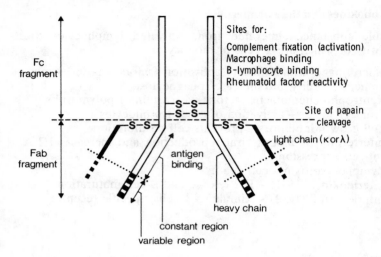

Figure 16.1 A diagram of an immunoglobulin molecule. Two identical light and identical heavy chains are shown. The Fab fragment hinges on the Fc fragment. The flexibility of the antigen binding site is dependent upon the interchain disulphide (– S –S –) bridges

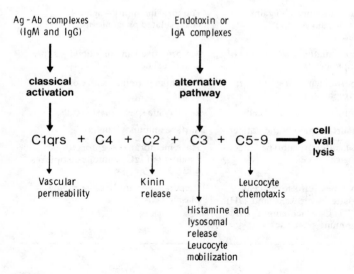

Figure 16.2 The complement cascade

Functions of the immunoglobulins

IgG – distributed in blood, interstitial fluids and across the placenta

1. The major Ig of the secondary immune response
2. Binds complement
3. Neutralizes soluble toxins

IgM – predominantly intravascular. Made of 5 Ig sub-units. Has 10 binding sites

1. The major Ig of the primary immune response
2. Activates complement hence producing lysis of foreign cells
3. Links particulate antigens for phagocytosis and agglutination
4. The blood group antigens are IgM
5. Many of the natural antibodies to bacteria are IgM

IgA – much present in the gut wall and respiratory tract

1. Major role in protection of mouth, gut and bronchi
2. High concentration in colostrum

IgD – possesses some of the properties of IgG but precise functions are unknown

IgE – Low serum concentration. Adheres to cell surfaces

1. Immediate hypersensitivity reactions such as hay fever
2. Possibly aid in defence against helminths

Functions of complement

1. C3b binds to cells and can then be bound to macrophages (immune adherence) allowing phagocytosis. This is the most important property
2. Chemotaxis for polymorphs $\left.\right\}$ via C3a and C5a
3. Histamine release – anaphylatoxin
4. C5b6789 causes cell lysis

Types of immune reaction

Type I.   Anaphylactic – may be localized as in hay fever or infrequently systemic as in anaphylactic shock. IgE mediated. Atopic diseases – hay fever, asthma

Type II. Cytotoxic – antibody directed against surface compo-
nents of a cell as in autoimmune haemolytic anaemia
(Coombs' test) and the very rare anti-GBM disease.
Mediated by IgM, IgG

Type III. Immune complex – deposition of antigen and antibody
tissues leading to inflammation. Examples – many
glomerulonephritides, rheumatoid arthritis, SLE,
serum sickness, lepromatous leprosy

Type IV. Delayed hypersensitivity – T-cells stimulated by antigen. Example – intracellular antigens such as viral
infections, tuberculosis, tuberculous leprosy

Type V.   Stimulating antibodies – some IgG antibodies stimulate
the cells against which they are directed. Examples –
anti-TSH receptor antibody in Graves' disease

Type VI. Antibody-dependent cell-mediated cytotoxicity
(ADCC) – K-cells in the presence of excess antibody
may be cytotoxic to cells coated with specific antigen.
Examples – defence against schistosomiasis, aspects of
autoimmunity and tumour rejection

Types II and III are complement dependent – that is, complement
has to be consumed for these two immune reactions to occur.

Methods of assessing cellular immunity

1. Skin testing – delayed hypersensitivity using PPD, *Candida*,
   streptokinase-streptodornase, staphylococcal or mumps antigens
2. T-cell counts   ⎫ chiefly of use in defining
   the main effector cells ⎬ malignancies of the immune system
3. B-cell counts   ⎭ and primary immunodeficiencies
4. Analysis of T-cell subsets – helper or suppres-
   sor cells
5. Proliferative response to antigens or mitogens
6. Migration inhibitory factors
7. Mixed lymphocyte culture
8. Antibody dependent cell-mediated cytotoxicity   infrequently
9. Macrophages and neutrophils   required

   i.   binding and ingestion of particles
   ii. degranulation
   iii. bactericidal activity
   iv. chemotaxis

Skin responses to external antigens

Type I.   Prick test – weal and erythematous flare within a few minutes of contact with antigen. Lasts not more than 20 minutes. Specific IgE mediated

Type III. Intradermal injection – immediate wealing which wanes in 1–2 hours then followed at 4–5 hours by a soft ill-defined oedematous reaction maximal at 5–7 hours and resolving within 24 hours

Type IV. Tuberculin test – an area of inflammatory oedema not less than 5 mm in diameter with surrounding erythema maximal at 2–4 days after the intradermal injection. Delayed hypersensitivity; T-cell mediated

Atopy

A familial tendency to develop abnormal hypersensitivity to common antigens. High concentrations of specific IgE antibody. Examples – hay fever, allergic rhinitis, extrinsic allergic asthma, gut cow's milk allergy of infants, infantile eczema.

PREDISPOSING FACTORS – often none

1. Immunoglobulin deficiencies, especially IgA
2. Lack of T-suppressor cells capable of ending IgE production
3. Mucosal defects as in cystic fibrosis

Common causes of immune complex disease
TABLE 16.3

Type	Antigens	Disease
Autoimmune	Nucleic acids	Systemic lupus erythematosus (SLE)
	IgG	Rheumatoid disease (arthritis)
Exogenous antigens	Gliadin	Gluten sensitivity
	Micropolyspora faenei	Extrinsic allergic alveolitis
	Penicillin	
	Sulphonamides	serum sickness
	Procainamide	
	Hydralazine	SLE syndrome
Infections	Bacterial	Meningococcal infection
		Subacute bacterial endocarditis
	M. leprae	Erythema nodosa leprosum
	Protazoal	Malaria
		Schistosomiasis } nephritis
	Viral	Hepatitis B

Autoantibodies in organ-specific and systemic autoimmune diseases

TABLE 16.4

Organ specific	Autoantibody present	Detected by
1. Myasthenia gravis	Anti-acetylcholine receptor	RIA
2. Graves' disease	LATS or anti-TSH receptor Ab	RIA
3. Addison's disease	Anti-adrenal Ab	IF
4. Insulin-dependent diabetes	Islet cell Ab	IF
5. Idiopathic hypoparathyroidism	Ab to parathyroid cell Ag	IF
6. Primary biliary cirrhosis	Ab to mitochondrial Ag	IF
7. Pernicious anaemia	Ab to gastric parietal cells and B_{12} binding site of IF	IF
8. Autoimmune haemolytic anaemia	Anti-RBC Ab	Coombs' test
9. Autoimmune thrombocytopenic purpura	Anti-platelet Ab	IF
10. Goodpasture's syndrome	Anti-basement membrane	RIA
Systemic		
1. Rheumatoid arthritis	Rheumatoid factor	Sensitized – SRBC agglutination. Latex agglutination. RIA
2. Systemic lupus erythematosus	Antinuclear Ab (ANA)	IF
	Anti ds- and ss-DNA	Farr assay, RIA
	Anti-Sm Ab	Haemagglutination RIA
	Anti-lymphocyte Ab	IF, cytotoxicity
3. Mixed connective tissue disease (MCTD)	Anti-ribonucleoprotein (RNP) Ab	Haemagglutination

Key to autoantibody table

Ab = antibody
Ag = antigen
RIA = radioimmunoassay
IF = immunofluorescence

SRBC = sheep red blood cells
ds = double stranded
ss = single stranded

Classification of immunodeficiency diseases

TABLE 16.5 (nearly all rare)

	Laboratory findings
B-cell (antibody) disorders	
1. X-linked infantile hypogammaglobulinaemia	1. Very reduced IgG. No IgM, IgA, IgD, IgE 2. No circulating B-cells
2. Acquired hypogammaglobulinaemia	1. IgG <250 mg/dl, with reduction in all immunoglobulins 2. Normal B-cell count
3. Selective IgA deficiency	IgA <5 mg/dl
T-cell disorders	
1. Acquired immunodeficiency syndrome	see page 261
2. Congenital thymic aplasia – DiGeorge syndrome	1. Absent T-cell functions 2. Lymphopenia and reduced T-cell count
3. Chronic mucocutaneous candidiasis	Negative skin testing to *Candida* antigen
Combined B- and T-cell deficiencies	
1. Severe combined immunodeficiency	1. Absence of B- and T-cell immunity 2. Absence or marked reduction in B- and T-cell counts
2. Ataxia-telangiectasia	1. Various T-cell abnormalities 2. IgA deficiency in 50 per cent of patients
3. Immunodeficiency with recurrent infection, eczema, and thrombocytopenia	1. Thrombocytopenia 2. Decreased IgM, normal IgG 3. Increased IgA and IgE
Phagocytic dysfunction diseases	
1. Chronic granulomatous diseases	1. Absent NBT dye reduction 2. Impaired bactericidal activity 3. Hypergammaglobulinaemia
2. Chediak–Higashi syndrome	1. Reduced bactericidal ability 2. Giant lysosomes
Complement deficiencies	Deficiencies of various complement components which may be associated with SLE or mesangiocapillary glomerulonephritis

HLA antigens

The genetic information for the human leucocyte antigens (HLA) is located on the shorter arms of chromosome 6. Four loci have been identified (HLA-A, -B, -C and -D). Also D related (-DR) antigens are recognized which are either identical or very similar to those produced by the HLA-D locus. The whole of the HLA region is known as the major histocompatibility complex (MHC). The presence of some HLA antigens appears to permit the development of some diseases. For example, a young man having HLA-B27 is about 100 times more likely to develop ankylosing spondylitis than a similar individual who does not possess this antigen.

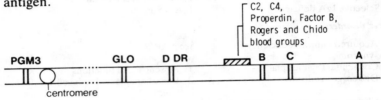

Short arm

Figure 16.3 The relative positions of loci in the HLA region on chromosome 6. The complement components C2, C4, Properdin, Factor B and two blood groups have structural genes in the region shown. In addition, phosphoglucomutase 3 (PGM3) and glyoxylase (GLO) enzymes are coded as shown

Haplotype – the combined genetic information (HLA haplotype) which an individual inherits from each parent with the corresponding HLA chromosomal region with its particular gene (allele) at each locus.

Linkage disequilibrium (allelic association) – the frequency of a haplotype for any three HLA antigens would be expected to be the product of the individual gene frequencies for the three alleles. The calculated permutations of HLA antigens exceed 300×10^6. Haplotype frequency is much more common than this. This phenomenon is called linkage disequilibrium. Some HLA genes are transmitted *en bloc* from generation to generation presumably by a reduction in the frequency of the normal process of genetic recombination during meiosis.

Relative risk – a measure of the strength of association between an HLA antigen and a disease is the relative risk ab/cd where a and c respectively represent the number of patients with and without the antigen and b and d the corresponding numbers for healthy controls. If there is no association the risk is 1.

Letter 'w' – this denotes an antigen which has been studied in International Workshops (w) but whose definition remains provisional; e.g. DRw8

Classification of diseases associated with HLA

TABLE 16.6 Idiopathic diseases (generally associated with A, B and C loci)

HLA	Disease	Relative risk
A3	Haemochromatosis	9
B27	Ankylosing spondylitis	90
B27	Reiter's arthritis	37
B27	Psoriatic arthritis	4.0
B27	Acute anterior uveitis	13
B35	de Quervain's sub-acute thyroiditis	14
Cw6	Psoriasis	13
B5	Behçet's disease	6
B2, B9	ALL – long survivors	unknown
B8	Hodgkin's disease – long survivors	unknown

TABLE 16.7 Immunological diseases (tend to be associated with -DR region)

HLA	Disease	Relative risk
DR2	Anti-GBM disease	16
	Multiple sclerosis	4
DR3	Myasthenia gravis – less likely to have a thymoma	3
	Graves' disease	5
	Sjögren's disease	10
	Chronic active hepatitis – not HBsAg hepatitis	7
	Idiopathic membranous glomerulonephritis	12
	Coeliac disease	11
	Systemic lupus erythematosus	6
	Dermatitis herpetiformis	15
	IDDM	4
DR4	IDDM	4
	Rheumatoid arthritis	4
DR5	Pernicious anaemia	5

Evidence of immunopathogenesis of rheumatoid arthritis

1. Hypergammaglobulinaemia
2. IgM rheumatoid factor in serum and synovial fluid
3. Circulating immune complexes in serum and synovial fluid
4. Immune complexes deposited in synovium
5. Activation of complement system
6. Lymphokines recoverable from synovium – T-cell activity
7. Association of RA with HLA–D4 and DR4

Evidence for immunopathogenesis of glomerulonephritis

1. Antigen needed (recognized in some) for initiation
2. Circulating immune complexes in serum
3. Immune complexes and complement components demonstrable in glomeruli
4. Activation of complement cascade
5. Resolution of acute nephritis if 'casual' antigen eradicated
6. Certain nephritides HLA – DR related

Indications for plasmaphoresis

Selected patients suffering from one of the following conditions which proves to be refractory to conventional treatment

HYPERVISCOSITY SYNDROME

1. Macroglobulinaemia
2. Myeloma

IMMUNE COMPLEX DISEASES

1. Systemic lupus erythematosus
2. Rapidly progressive glomerulonephritis
3. Essential cryoglobulinaemia

ANTIBODY MEDIATED DISEASE

1. Myasthenia gravis
2. Rhesus iso-immunization
3. Idiopathic thrombocytopenic purpura
4. Goodpasture's syndrome

Graft–versus–host disease

DEFINITION

An attack by the donor's immunologically reactive lymphocytes against the 'foreign' antigens of the host.

GVH may be acute or chronic. Skin, gastrointestinal tract and liver are the main targets. Mortality may be up to 75 per cent. Opportunistic infections are not infrequent.

Acquired immune deficiency syndrome (AIDS)

INTRODUCTION

A systemic infection, invariably fatal, primarily affecting homosexuals caused by the Human Immunodeficiency Virus (HIV) usually transmitted by buggery but also by bisexual intercourse, infected needles in drug addicts, blood and blood products. Severe immunodeficiency develops due to loss of T-helper/inducer cells. Patients usually die of *Pneumocystis carinii* pneumonia or an aggressive form of Kaposi's sarcoma or both. AIDS is spreading exponentially but neither prevalence nor incidence is known. Those infected with HIV develop either AIDS, AIDS-related complex (ARC) or persistent generalized lymphadenopathy (PLG). The precise relationships between AIDS, ARC and PLG have yet to be clearly defined. Patients with antibodies against HIV do not necessarily eventually develop AIDS. Clinical spectrum of AIDS is enlarging. Median survival after diagnosis of AIDS is 9–30 months.

IMMUNOLOGY

HIV binds to T-helper/inducer cells (CD4) and antigen recognition cells which are then unable to function adequately. No activated killer cells are available to assist in host defence and thus allow repeated infections. Why *P. carinii* infections and Kaposi's sarcoma predominate is unknown. In the late stages of AIDS, immunoglobulin concentrations fall. A poor prognosis is associated with a decreasing titre of antibodies to HIV core protein.

Shortly after infection there is a rise T-cytotoxic/suppressor (CD8) cells and tests of lymphocyte function start to become abnormal. As PLG and ARC develop the fall in CD4 cells is inexorable. Intracellular killing of bacteria by lymphocytes is impaired and Type IV reactions are lost. Virus replication (reverse transcriptase) occurs in dividing CD4 cells.

TRANSMISSION OF HIV

1. Sexual intercourse – anal or vaginal
2. Contaminated needles

   i.   intravenous drug abusers
   ii. needle stick injuries

3. Mother to child

   i.   *in utero*
   ii. perhaps via breast milk

4. Donation of

   i.   semen
   ii. solid organs
   iii. skin

Particularly infectious fluids are blood, semen and vaginal secretions.

CLINICAL FEATURES

AIDS has been diagnosed in

1. Homosexuals – the vast majority of European and American cases
2. Intravenous drug addicts – moderate numbers
3. Bisexual males – modest numbers
4. Prostitutes – male and female – variable numbers
5. Patients who have received blood or blood products – very small numbers
6. Any combination of the above lifestyles leads to much higher rates of HIV antibody presence.

Acute HIV seroconversion includes a glandular fever like syndrome with an excellent immediate outlook. For those who develop PLG, biopsy is indicated in those with

1. Asymmetrical node enlargement
2. Painful nodes
3. Sudden increase in size
4. Hilar lymphadenopathy

with or without constitutional symptoms

CONSTITUTIONAL SYMPTOMS INCLUDE

1. Fever for >1 month
2. Diarrhoea for >1 month
3. Loss of >10 per cent of ideal body weight

Many different skin diseases of an infectious nature may develop.

Haematological abnormalities include

1. Lymphopenia
2. Neutropenia
3. Thrombocytopenia – usually moderate
4. Anaemia – usually not <10 g/dl

A combination of constitutional symptoms, skin or mucosal infection with haematological abnormalities (ARC) appears to predict the later development of AIDS.

AIDS AND RELATED TUMOURS

1. Kaposi's sarcoma
2. Malignant lymphoma } chiefly in homosexuals

AIDS AND LUNG INFECTIONS

1. *P. carinii* – 85 per cent
2. Cytomegalovirus
3. Bacterial pneumonias – *Streptococcus pneumoniae* and *Haemophilus influenzae*
4. *Myobacterium kansaii* > *M. tuberculosis*
5. Fungi – infrequent.

Both malignant and lung complications are recorded in renal transplant recipients but very rarely – unlike AIDS.

AIDS AND THE GUT

1. Oral and oesophageal candidiasis
2. CMV and *Herpes simplex* ulcers – from mouth to anus
3. Diarrhoea common and unexplained
4. Hepatitis – atypical myobacteria, *Cryptococcus neoformans* or CMV
5. Hairy leukoplakia
6. Proctitis – HSV, *Neisseria gonorrhoeae* or *Chlamydia-trachomatis*
7. Recurrent anogenital warts

NEUROLOGICAL MANIFESTATIONS OF AIDS

1. Encephalitis – thought to be direct effect of HIV
2. Meningitis – main cause *C. neoformans*
3. Space occupying lesions – *Toxoplasma gondii* abscesses and other tumours
4. Demyelination – progressive multifocal; papovavirus
5. Retinitis – CMV most common
6. Myelopathy   } considered to be a direct
7. Peripheral neuropathy } effect of HIV

Chapter 17

Rheumatological and collagen-vascular diseases

Rheumatoid disease (arthritis; RA)

A systemic connective tissue disorder chiefly affecting joints in a peripheral symmetrical, non-suppurative chronic manner frequently combined with non-articular features. Morning stiffness is characteristic. Subcutaneous nodules, articular erosions and circulating rheumatoid factor are common. Women more than men. Affects 3–4 per cent of population. RA is associated with the MHC antigen Dw4.

PATHOLOGY

1. Oedematous, congested and hypertrophied synovium with prominent accumulation of plasma cells, lymphocytes and macrophages
2. Nodules with central fibrinoid necrosis and palisades of inflammatory cells on extensor surfaces
3. Vasculitis of small blood vessels especially the fingers

JOINTS

Most commonly affected are – wrists, proximal interphalangeal and metacarpophalangeal of hands, metatarso-phalangeal, knees. Less frequent – elbows, shoulders, tarsus, ankles, hips, neck, temporomandibular joints.

MAJOR RADIOLOGICAL FINDINGS

Sequential features

1. Soft tissue swelling
2. Juxta-articular osteoporosis – immobility
3. Erosions at joint margins – best seen in small joints of hands and radial or ulna styloids. A bad prognostic sign
4. Loss of joint-space – cartilage damage
5. Deformity of knees and elbows
6. Reabsorption of distal ends of clavicles
7. Subluxation of C1 on C2
8. Hip joints – protrusio acetabuli

Extra-articular features

1. Systemic – often prodromal
    i.   malaise
    ii. fever
    iii. myalgia
    iv. fatigue
    v.   weight loss

2. Skin
    i.   nodules – extensor surfaces at pressure points (common) associated with seropositivity
    ii. ruddy, cyanotic skin over small joints

3. Blood
    i.   anaemia – normochromic, normocytic
    ii.   anaemia – iron deficient; secondary to aspirin, NSAI drugs or steroids
    iii. Coombs positive anaemia
    iv.   IgM rheumatoid factor (RF) present in 80 per cent
    v.   ESR and C-reactive protein
    vi.   thrombocytopenia – gold therapy or Felty's syndrome
    vii. ANF positive in 20 per cent

4. RES
    i.   lymphadenopathy – common feature of active disease
    ii. splenomegaly
    iii. Felty's syndrome – spleen, RA and leucopenia

5. Vasculitis
    i.   nail fold and finger pulp infarcts
    ii. Raynaud's phenomenon
    iii. chronic leg ulcers

6. Lung
    i.   pleurisy at times with effusion – low glucose concentration
    ii. nodules
    iii. interstitial fibrosis – rare

7. Heart – pericarditis – often sub-clinical

8. Eye
    i.   keratoconjunctivitis sicca – the most common
    ii. scleritis or episcleritis
    iii. scleromalacia perforans – nodule involvement
    iv. drug effects – steroids particularly

9. Muscle – weakness and wasting are common
10. Psychology
    i.   depression
    ii. loss of appetite and interests
11. Neuropathy – frequent
    i.   entrapment – especially carpal tunnel syndrome
    ii. peripheral neuropathy
         (a) distal sensory – good prognosis
         (b) sensorimotor – bad prognosis
    iii. mononeuritis multiplex – rare
12. Kidney
    i.   proteinuria from gold or penicillamine therapy
    ii. amyloid is a rare complication (but less so in JCA)

Common deformities of RA

1. Deformity, subluxation, ulnar deviation, swan neck and boutonnière deformities
2. Tendon rupture
3. Ulnar nerve compression – at the elbow
4. Baker's cyst rupture
5. 'Z' thumbs
6. Pyoarthritis
7. Flexion contractures – knees and elbows
8. Median nerve compression (carpal tunnel)
9. Fixed wrists
10. Bowed knees
11. Valgus ankles (turned outward)
12. Wide, splayed forefoot with subluxation of toes
13. Cord compression due to cervical or odontoid peg subluxation
14. Crico-arytenoid involvement causing hoarseness or obstruction

Presenting factors in RA

POOR PROGNOSIS

1. Nodules
2. Polyarticular presentation
3. Vasculitis or other systemic lesions
4. Early bony erosions
5. High titre rheumatoid factor >1 in 512
6. Positive DNA binding

GENERAL PROGNOSIS

For a new patient attending a hospital outpatient clinic

1. 20 per cent permanent remission without any residue
2. 25 per cent permanent remission with mild residue
3. 45 per cent persistent activity with variable progressive deformity
4. 10 per cent progression to complete disability

Juvenile chronic arthritis (JCA; Still's disease)

MAJOR FEATURES

1. Onset before age of 12 years
2. Girls more than boys
3. Large joint involvement
4. Radiological erosions within 12 months
5. Early muscle wasting
6. Prominent systemic features – extra-articular features of RA are common

    i.   transient rash
    ii. fever
    iii. lymphadenopathy
    iv. splenomegaly
    v.   amyloid more frequent than in RA

MODES OF ONSET

1. Acute febrile – young children; systemic features; 25 per cent develop progressive disease
2. Polyarticular – progressive, worst prognosis
3. Monoarticular – insidious onset; mild features; best prognosis

Systemic lupus erythematosus (SLE)

DEFINITION

A non-organ specific auto-immune disease which may affect any organ, but primarily involving blood vessels, serosal surfaces and joints. More common in women than men, West Indians than Europeans. An association with B8 and DR3 tissue types.

GENERAL PATHOLOGICAL FEATURES

1. Fibrinoid necrosis – joints, kidneys, and lungs
2. Deposition of immune complexes – dermal-epidermal junction, glomerular basement membranes, choroid plexus
3. Haemotoxylin bodies – involved tissues

IMMUNOLOGICAL FEATURES

1. Circulating antibodies to double stranded DNA ⎫
2. Circulating immune complexes   ⎬ all maximal during exacer-
3. Complement consumption – CH50, C4 and C3   ⎪ bation of the disease
   reduced   ⎭
4. Reduced cell-mediated immune responses
5. Coombs' positive haemolytic anaemia in some
6. Lymphocytotoxins
7. Cryoglobulins

Clinical features of SLE

1. Musculo-articular – occur in virtually all patients

   i.   arthritis or arthralgia ⎫ common
   ii. myalgia or myositis   ⎭
   iii. deforming arthritis ⎫ infrequent
   iv. bone changes   ⎭
        (a) avascular necrosis
        (b) erosions

2. Cutaneous – occurs in 80 per cent of patients

   i.   vasculitis   ⎫
   ii. facial rash – 'butterfly' ⎬ common (60–70 per cent)
   iii. alopecia   ⎭
   iv. Raynaud's phenomenon   ⎫
   v.   mouth ulcers   ⎬ about 30 per cent of patients
   vi. photosensitivity – a precipitant of SLE ⎭

3. Fever – up to 80 per cent of patients; usually with other signs

4. Neurological system* – occurs in up to 60 per cent of patients
    i.   depression
    ii. psychosis
    iii. fits
    iv. variety of long tract, cranial nerve or basal ganglia manifestations
    v.   peripheral neuropathy – rare

5. Renal* – about 50 per cent of patients
    i.   proteinuria or nephrotic state ⎤ manifestations of renal
    ii. haematuria   ⎬ lupus – usually diffuse
    iii. decline in GFR   ⎦ proliferative or focal nephritides

6. Lungs – about 50 per cent of patients
    i.   pleurisy
    ii. effusions – exudate with a normal glucose concentration
    iii. non-bacterial pneumonia
    iv. elevated diaphragms ⎤ rare, but Dco reduced in many
    v.   fibrosis   ⎬ SLE patients without apparent
                             ⎦ lung involvement

7. Heart – involved in about 40 per cent of patients
    i.   pericarditis – frequent but usually sub-clinical
    ii. conduction defects – rare

HAEMATOLOGICAL FEATURES OF SLE

1. Lymphopenia
2. Leucopenia – WBC $<4.5 \times 10^9/\ell$ ⎤ frequently present
3. Anaemia – normochromic, normocytic ⎦
4. Anaemia – haemolytic, moderately frequent
5. Thrombocytopenia – mild and common
6. Lymphocyte cytotoxic antibodies – common

DRUGS IMPLICATED IN DRUG-SLE

1. Anticonvulsants – phenytoin, primidone ⎤ Result tends to be
2. Isoniazid   ⎥ dose dependent
3. Chlorpromazine   ⎥ and reversible
4. Oral contraceptives may exacerbate   ⎬ upon withdrawing
   pre-existing SLE   ⎥ the drug. Renal
5. Hydralazine   ⎥ and CNS
6. Procainamide   ⎦ involvement rare

* Neurological and renal involvements are serious and potential fatal complications of SLE.

PROGNOSIS OF SLE

This is changing and improving. Bad prognostic factors

1. Diffuse, drug-resistant proliferative
   nephritis
2. Severe recurrent CNS involvement

} 5-year survival about 50 per cent

A comparison of RA and SLE

TABLE 17.1

	RA	SLE
Age at onset	All ages	15–40
Sex incidence (F:M)	3:1	9:1
Arthritis	Prominent	Mild
Erosions	Common	Rare
Fever	Rare	Common
Rashes	Rare	Common
Nodules	Common	Rare
Renal involvement	Rare	50 per cent of cases
CNS involvement	Very rare	60 per cent of cases
Haemolytic anaemia	Very rare	Fairly common
DNA binding	Up to 5 per cent	100 per cent in active phase
Rheumatoid factor	70–80 per cent	Up to 40 per cent
Serum complement	Normal	Reduced in active phase
Circulating immune complexes	Present in joints	Up to 100 per cent in active phase

Sjögren's syndrome

1. Keratoconjunctivitis sicca – dry eyes ⎫ sicca syndrome
2. Xerostomia – dry mouth   ⎬ (KCS)
3. Connective tissue disease

   i.   seropositive RA – usually ⎫
   ii. scleroderma   ⎪
   iii. SLE   ⎬ secondary Sjögren syndrome
   iv. Hashimoto's thyroiditis   ⎭

PATHOLOGY

Inflammation, infiltration by plasma cells and lymphocytes with later fibrosis occurring in mucus secreting glands.

IMMUNOLOGICAL FEATURES

IgM rheumatoid factor is present in virtually all patients with KCS. The ANF is positive in about 70 per cent, while antibodies to DNA may be found in 10 per cent. In addition, antibodies are found (in descending order of frequency) with activity against salivary duct cells, gastric parietal, thyroglobulin, thyroid microsomal, mitochondrial and smooth muscle cells. The serum concentration of IgM is often raised.

Sjögren's syndrome may be associated with a large number of different clinical manifestations. The best known are

1. Liver disease – primary biliary cirrhosis and chronic active hepatitis
2. Renal disease – renal tubular acidosis; 25 per cent of patients with Sjögren's syndrome
3. Raynaud's phenomenon – in 30 per cent of patients
4. Lymphoreticular neoplasia

Polymyalgia rheumatica and giant cell arteritis

DEFINITION

Aching girdle pains, stiffness, raised ESR. Elderly patients. Females more than males. A proportion of these patients have biopsy proof of giant cell arteritis and a smaller proportion have clinical giant cell arteritis. No specific or unique diagnostic test available.

FEATURES

1. Myalgia – stiff and slightly tender muscles
2. Systemic features – mild fever, weight loss, anaemia
3. Arterial symptoms – tender arteries of scalp, jaw claudication, tongue pain, sudden blindness

Features 1–2 may occur without any of the features 3, and vice versa.

Polyarteritis nodosa (PAN)

Inflammation of medium sized and small blood vessels occurs chiefly affecting the skin, lung and kidney. There is infarction distal to the panarteritis. Aetology in unknown. 5-year survival – 50 per cent.

MAIN FEATURES

1. Fever, weight loss, skin lesions
2. Haematuria, proteinuria, rapid decline in GFR
3. Accelerated phase hypertension
4. Asthma or focal lung infiltrates
5. Muscle pain, tenderness and wasting
6. Acute abdomen
7. CNS lesions

} all due to arterial inflammation and distal infarction

Progressive systemic sclerosis–PSS (Scleroderma)

DEFINITION

Widespread sclerosis affecting skin, gut, muscle, heart, kidney and lung. Raynaud's phenomenon almost invariable. Women more often affected than men. Progressive, fatal, rare.

MAIN FEATURES

1. Skin
   i.   taut, tethered, hands, neck and chest
   ii. loss of mobility
   iii. subcutaneous calcification in fingers
   iv. Raynaud's phenomenon

2. Gut
   i.   oesophagus – dysphagia and reflux oesophagitis – common
   ii. small gut – cramps, fullness, malabsorption
   iii. Sjögren's syndrome

3. Musculo-skeletal – myopathy of shoulder girdle – 40 per cent of patients

4. Heart – myocardial fibrosis and conduction defects; often asymptomatic

5. Kidney – renal failure may develop in months. Severe hypertension

6. Lung – involvement occurs in 40 per cent of patients. May be asymptomatic
   i.   fibrosis
   ii. honeycombing
   iii. infections – including reflux pneumonitis

CREST syndrome

1. Calcinosis
2. Raynaud's phenomenon
3. Oesophagus
4. Sclerodactyly
5. Telangiectasia

This appears to be a sub-group of patients with scleroderma who develop prominent cutaneous features but minimal or no visceral disease

Mixed connnective tissue disease (MCTD)

DEFINITION

A condition which has features of SLE, polymyositis, scleroderma or RA to differing extents. Diagnosed serologically

1. Extractable nuclear antigen antibodies – ENA
2. ENA antibodies contain anti-ribonucleoprotein antibodies – RNP
3. The presence of anti-RNP antibodies appears to confer a much better prognosis than that of PSS

Seronegative arthropathies

DEFINITION

Inflammatory arthritides in which IgM rheumatoid factor is *not* present. The main diseases of this group are

1. Ankylosing spondylitis – 90 per cent have HLA-B27
2. Psoriatic arthritis
3. Reiter's disease
4. Colitic arthritis
5. Behçet's syndrome

Each of these conditions may develop features similar to, or identical with, those of ankylosing spondylitis. HLA B27 is more frequently present than in control populations

Ankylosing spondylitis

An erosive arthropathy with bony ankylosis primarily affecting the S-I joints and spine. Incidence similar to that of RA. Proximal limb joints also involved. Restricted movements of spine and thoracic cage. Male to female ratio 9:1 but now being diagnosed more frequently in women. Third decade onset.

COMPLICATIONS

1. Non-granulomatous anterior uveitis – up to 40 per cent
2. Ulcerative colitis – 10 per cent
3. Apical pulmonary fibrosis – 1 per cent
4. Aortic incompetence, cardiomegaly and conduction defects – up to 10 per cent

RADIOLOGY

1. Sacro-iliitis leading to bony ankylosis
2. Squaring of vertebral bodies
3. Bony bridges between vertebrae – syndesmophytes or 'bamboo spine'
4. Erosion and later fusion of symphysis pubis

PROGNOSIS

Progressive disease in many.

Psoriatic arthritis

Erosive arthritis; no nodules. Terminal interphalangeal finger joints, I–P joint of thumb, and I–P joints of toes. S–I joints may become involved. Equal sex incidence. Nail pitting in 60–80 per cent of patients. Occurs in about 20% of patients with psoriasis.

PROGNOSIS

Progressive but less severe than rheumatoid arthritis.

Reiter's syndrome

Recurrent attacks of polyarthritis in legs, S–I joints and spine, associated with non-gonococcal urethritis or dysentry – reactive arthritis. 98 per cent males.

FEATURES

1. Arthritis and conjunctivitis – 30 per cent; 1–2 weeks after urethritis
2. Circinate balanitis – 30 per cent in the uncircumcised
3. Keratoderma blenorrhagica – 10 per cent, usually soles of feet
4. Nail lesions
5. Transient painless buccal ulcers
6. Anterior uveitis in 30–50 per cent of those who progress to chronic arthritis

PROGNOSIS

Was considered to be self-limiting in the majority. It has been found that disease activity is present in 80 per cent 5 years from outset.

Colitic arthritis

1. Of patients with ulcerative colitis or Crohn's disease 10 per cent develop a peripheral seronegative inflammatory arthritis
2. Of patients with ankylosing spondylitis 10 per cent develop ulcerative colitis

Behçet's syndrome

Rare

1. Mouth ulcers – 100 per cent
2. Genital ulcers – 90 per cent
3. Arthritis of large weight bearing joints – 60 per cent
4. Erythema nodosum – 25 per cent
5. Thrombophlebitis – 20 per cent
6. Anterior uveitis – 10 per cent

Crystal deposition diseases

Gout

DEFINITION

A disease of men with high serum acid concentrations (>0.5 mmol/ℓ) although asymptomatic hyperuricaemia is quite common. Crystals of monosodium urate monohydrate are deposited in joints and other tissues.

Causes of hyperuricaemia

1. Decreased renal excretion
   i. primary gout – in the presence of a normal GFR
   ii. chronic renal failure – but gout is very infrequent

2. Drugs
   i. thiazides
   ii. salicylates
   iii. probenicid
   iv. sulphinpyrazone } low dose
   v. ethambutol
   vi. pyrazinamide

   but hyperuricaemia is unusual and gout an infrequent side effect of these drugs

3. Reduction in fractional urate clearance

    i.   diabetic ketoacidosis
    ii. starvation, vomiting, alcohol 'binges'
    iii. hypertension
    iv. hypothyroidism
    v.   toxaemia of pregnancy

4. Increased production of uric acid

    i.   lymphoproliferative disorders* including
         (a) chronic lymphatic leukaemia
         (b) Hodgkin's
         (c) lymphosarcoma
    ii. myeloproliferative disorders* including
         (a) chronic myeloid leukaemia
         (b) primary and secondary polycythaemias
    iii. haemolytic states
         (a) haemoglobinopathies
         (b) pernicious anaemia
    iv. carcinomatosis and multiple myeloma
    v.   concentrated fructose infusions
    vi. severe exfoliative psoriasis

5. Increased purine synthesis *(de novo)*

    All rare obscure conditions

Clinical features of acute gout

1. Often begins in the great toe joint in men aged 30 or more years
2. Usually peripheral joints but can be any joint
3. Post-pubertal men and less frequently post-menopausal women affected
4. May be provoked by

    i.   trauma, including surgery
    ii. severe dieting – or starvation illness
    iii. excess alcohol
    iv. beginning allopurinol, B_{12} or uricosuric drugs
5. The affected joint is

    i.   hot
    ii. red
    iii. swollen with shiny skin
    iv. excruciatingly painful

* Hyperuricaemia most likely to occur when cytotoxic drugs are begun

Chronic tophaceous gout

Uncommon

1. A consequence of recurrent acute attacks
2. Asymmetrical joint swelling
3. Tophi – periarticular tissues, ear cartilage, tendon sheaths and bursae
4. Chronic interstitial nephritis due to urate deposition

Pyrophosphate arthropathy (pseudogout)

Shedding of calcium pyrophosphate dihydrate into the joint space.

FEATURES

1. Knees of elderly patients most commonly affected
2. May have recurrent acute arthritis
3. May be chronic with calcium deposition in the joint cartilage – chondrocalcinosis
4. May complicate chronic hypercalcaemias

Differentiation between urate and pyrophosphate crystals

TABLE 17.2

	Monosodium urate	Pyrophosphate
Length	2–10 μm	1–10 μm
Shape	Rods or crystals	Similar but may be shorter or thicker
Birefringence under polarized light	Strong negative	Weak positive

Unusual or rare arthropies

1. Viral – the following infections may be complicated by a short-lived arthropy
    i.   rubella – the most common
    ii. mumps
    iii. chickenpox
    iv. hepatitis B
    v.   infectious mononucleosis
    vi. arboviruses

2. Bacterial
    i. *Salmonella* and *Shigella* – arthropathy
    ii. *Yersinia enterocolitica* – reactive arthropathy, occasionally Reiter's syndrome
    iii. any bacterium – gonococcal becoming frequent
    iv. *Myobacterium tuberculosis* – immigrants and elderly, chiefly
    v. meningococcal infection – occurs in medium sized joints several days after infection

3. Endocrine diseases
    i. acromegaly – in 50 per cent of patients, due to cartilage overgrowth
    ii. hypothyroidism ⎫
    iii. hyperparathyroidism ⎬ very rare

4. Metabolic disorders
    i. haemochromatosis and Wilson's disease ⎫
    ii. hyperlipidaemias – especially Frederickson Type II ⎬ rare
    iii. ochronosis ⎪
    iv. Fabry's disease ⎭

5. Miscellaneous
    i. malignancy – including hypertrophic pulmonary osteoarthropathy and synovitis in patients with acute leukaemia
    ii. sarcoid
    iii. familial Mediterranean fever
    iv. haemophilia
    v. polychondritis
    vi. neuropathic joints

Chapter 18

Skin diseases

Definitions of morphological terms

Macule. A flat lesion without change in surface marking or texture.
Papule. A circumscribed palpable elevation or thickening of epidermis or upper dermis.
Plaque. A palpable mass >1 cm in diameter caused by oedema or infiltration into dermis or subcutaneous tissue.

Common dermatoses

Numbers 1–5 are the most common

1. Psoriasis – dominant transmission. Red patches with silvery scales. Predilection for extensor surfaces. Fluctuating course
2. Eczema – inflammatory disorder. Chiefly involves the epidermis. In the acute stage – oedema, exudation and crusting. In the chronic stage – hyperplasia and hyperkeratosis
   i.   atopic – begins in early life
   ii. seborrhoeic – predilection for skin with a high sebaceous density
   iii. chronic – common; regresses if scratching stops
   iv. stasis – as in chronic venous stasis; topical applications have to be excluded
3. Acne – disease of sebaceous glands with follicular papules, pustules, blackheads and scars
   i.   adolescent
   ii. drug induced – corticosteroids, androgens, chlorpromazine, iodides
4. Urticarias – focal oedema of dermis due to a transient increase in capillary permeability
   i.   chronic idiopathic – F > M; peak incidence 20–40 years
   ii. hereditary angioedema – C1 esterase deficiency
   iii. physical – pressure, cold, heat and solar

5. Skin cancer
   i.   basal cell epithelioma (rodent ulcer) – locally malignant
   ii. squamous cell carcinoma – tumour of the keratinizing epidermis, usually of sun-exposed skin
   iii. malignant melanoma – tumour of the melanocyte cell series. Usually fatal
6. Ichthyosis – genetic and acquired. Characterized by a widespread scaly skin
7. Lichen planus – spontaneously waxing and waning disease of skin and mucous membrane with blue papules and white striae

Diffuse changes in skin colour

1. Cyanosis – peripheral and central
2. Pale – anaemia; usually $<8\,\text{g/d}\ell$ before detectable
3. Yellow to yellow-green – jaundice
4. Polycythaemia – deep red/blue
5. Pale lemon – Addisonian (pernicious) anaemia
6. Muddy yellow/brown – chronic haemodialysis patients
7. Advanced chronic disease – Addisonian-type pigmentation
8. Cushing's disease – nearly always iatrogenic
9. Haemochromatosis – slate-grey
10. Addison's disease – pale with palmar pigmentation
11. Carotenaemia – yellow
12. Ochronosis (alkaptanuria) – blue-black; cartilage especially
13. Mepacrine therapy – yellow
14. Nelson's syndrome – a deep tan
15. Chronic arsenic poisoning

rare

Industrial skin diseases

A very wide range of chemicals is involved

1. Contact dermatitis
   i. due to irritants
   ii. due to allergies
2. Industrial acne
3. Vinyl chloride disease
4. Depigmentation – adhesives workers
5. Skin cancer
6. Fluoride spots
7. Chrome ulcers

Causes of pruritus

DEFINITION

Sensation which provokes the desire to scratch.

1. Chronic cholestasis – typically primary biliary cirrhosis
2. Neoplasia – especially Hodgkin's disease
3. Allergic drug reactions
4. Advanced chronic renal failure – particularly dialysis patients
5. Heroin addicts
6. Psychological
7. Endocrine – hyper- and hypothyroidism; occasionally
8. Polycythaemia or iron deficiency

Vitiligo

DEFINITION

Sharply defined roughly symmetrical patches of depigmentation due to destruction of melanocytes. Chiefly affecting backs of hands and arms, face and neck, axillae, eyelids and genitalia.

CAUSES

1. Idiopathic
2. Associated disorders
   i.   hyperthyroidism
   ii. pernicious anaemia
   iii. late onset diabetes   anti-thyroglobulin, parietal
   iv. gastric cancer, melanoma cell and smooth muscle
   v. alopecia areata   antibodies found in varying
   vi. Addison's disease – rare   numbers in these patients
   vii. myxoedema

Severe pruritus secondary to skin disease

1. Scabies, insect bites, pediculosis
2. Eczema
3. Urticaria
4. Dermatitis herpetiformis – uncommon
5. Lichen planus
6. 'Prickly heat' – miliaria rubra

Drug induced pigmentation

1. Prolonged high dose chlorpromazine – generalized slate-grey pigmentation

2. Contraceptive pill – chloasma, irregular hyperpigmentation of the face, as in pregnancy
3. Topical drugs – hyper- and hypomelanization
4. Prolonged busulphan (for CML) – generalized pigmentation
5. ACTH – synthetic and endogenous; via its MSH activity
6. Chloroquine

Possible skin responses to drugs

For brevity, examples are not given

1. Exanthamata – the most common form
2. Urticarial – penicillins, sulphonamides, salicylates, phenothiazines are the most common causes
3. Purpura – gold, carbinazole
4. Photosensitivity – sulphonamides, chlorpropamide, nalidixic acid, griseofulvin
5. Eczema
6. Pigmentation – *see* above
7. Fixed eruptions – phenolphthalein
8. Bullous eruptions
9. Exfoliative dermatitis
10. Erythema nodosum

Blisters

DEFINITION

A blister is an elevated circumscribed lesion filled with serum and cells. Blister <0.5 cm diameter is a vesicle, larger blisters are called bullae.

1. Friction, pressure, frostbite
2. UV light sensitivity – especially in fair children
3. Drugs – tetracycline, sulphonamides, phenothiazines, thiazides, nalidixic acid, barbiturate overdose
4. Contact dermatitis – wide range of possible chemicals
5. Pompholyx – recurrent eczematoid interdigital itching and bullae
6. Fixed drug eruptions – phenolphthalein, sulphonamides, barbiturates, quinine
7. Dermatitis herpetiformis – severe itching, gluten sensitivity in 25 per cent of cases
8. Stevens–Johnson syndrome – severe erythema multiforme
9. Toxic epidermal necrolysis: adults, usually drug related ⎫
10. Pemphigus vulgaris – patients 40–60 years of age   ⎬ rare
11. Bullous pemphigoid – patients 60–80 years of age   ⎭

12. Viral
    i.   herpes simplex – 'cold sores'
    ii. herpes zoster – early phase of shingles

Alopecia

1. Follicular destruction
    i.   SLE – quite common in this disease
    ii. lichen planus, psoriasis
    iii. inflammatory – pyogenic, fungal, X-irradiation
2. Follicular dysfunction
    i.   older men and women
    ii. severe illness – loss of growing phase (anagen) follicles
    iii. severe malnutrition – same reason as in ii. above
    iv. alopecia areata – discrete patches of hair loss
    v.   drugs
        (a) cyclophosphamide
        (b) corticosteroids – particularly if topically applied
        (c) heparin – haemodialysis patients; coumarin derivatives
        (d) X-irradiation
3. Fibre fracture
    i.   trauma – habit, heating irons and chemicals
    ii. Menke's kinky hair disease – very rare; genetic defect of
         copper metabolism
4. Genetic – male-pattern baldness

Hypertrichosis

Growth of hair at sites not normally hairy

1. Racial
2. Endocrine – all rare
    i.   Cushing's syndrome
    ii. acromegaly
    iii. adreno-genital syndrome
    iv. precocious puberty
    v.   virilizing ovarian tumours
3. Drugs
    i.   corticosteroid – exogenous and endogenous ⎤
    ii. minoxidil and diazoxide   ⎥ fairly
    iii. antiepileptics   ⎥ common
    iv. anabolic steroids   ⎦
4. Psychological – anorexia nervosa

Nail conditions

Normal growth rate: fingernails 1 cm in 3 months; toe nails 1 cm in 12 months

1. Slow growth – many unrelated diseases
2. Clubbing – pulmonary osteoarthropathy, thyroid acropathy
3. Koilonychia – iron deficiency
4. Pallor – liver disease and other causes of hypoalbuminaemia; *see* page 70
5. Splinter haemorrhages – injury, vasculitis, psoriasis and SBE (the least common of these four causes)
6. Raynaud's phenomenon – may rarely be complicated by *Candida* infection and secondary nail dystrophy

Recurrent oral ulceration

1. Aphthous ulcers
2. Ulcerative colitis – identical to aphthous ulcers
3. Behçet's syndrome – larger than aphthous ulcers
4. Malabsorption syndromes
5. Crohn's disease
6. Coeliac disease – relationship debated
7. Systemic and discoid lupus – infrequent

Causes of red scaly rash

TABLE 18.1

Localized	Widespread
Psoriasis	Psoriasis
Eczema	Eczema
Fixed drug eruption	Resolving exanthemata – e.g. measles
Ringworm	Pityriasis rosea
Lichen simplex	Pityriasis versicolor

Pyoderma gangrenosum

1. Inflammatory bowel disease
2. Myeloma
3. Leukaemias and myelofibrosis
4. Fifty per cent have no associated conditions

Skin signs of chronic liver disease

1. Colour – greenish-yellow in prolonged icterus, yellow when jaundiced – grey-blue in haemochromatosis (rare; melanin deposition)
2. Vascule signs
    i.   spider naevi – upper half of body; common
    ii. liver palms – thena and hypothena eminences, pulps of finger; common but not specific
    iii. purpura and bruising – vitamin K deficiency; an advanced sign
    iv. caput medusa – occurs in portal hypertension; very rare
3. Hands
    i.   liver palms
    ii. leuconychia – impaired albumin synthesis
    iii. Dupuytren's contracture – non-specific
    iv. clubbing – rare
4. Endocrine abnormalities: presumably all related to excess oestrogen
    i.   testicular atrophy – mainly in alcoholics; common
    ii. gynaecomastia – mainly in alcoholic liver disease
    iii. acne – upper part of body
5. Skin changes
    i.   thin skin – veins more prominent
    ii. loss of pubic hair – common
    iii. body hair fine and lustreless
    iv. vitiligo – in chronic active and primary biliary cirrhosis
6. Miscellaneous
    i.   pruritus – with prolonged cholestasis
    ii. xanthomata – infrequent

Skin signs in chronic renal failure

1. Colour – pale, muddy yellow, persistent sun-tan, all best seen in haemodialysis patients
2. Pruritus – generalized scratch marks; common
3. Dryness – shins particularly; not frequent
4. Associated conditions
    i.   rash of SLE
    ii. changes of scleroderma   } rare
    iii. partial lipodystrophy

Skin signs of endocrine diseases

1. Hyperthyroidism – common
    i.   skin – warm and sweaty
    ii.   vitiligo ⎫
    iii. alopecia ⎬ in about 10 per cent of cases
    iv.   hair – normal or fine
    v.   pretibial myxoedema – rare
2. Hypothyroidism – common
    i.   skin – pale, coarse, puffy, scaly, cold and dry
    ii.   hair – loss on eyebrows and at times the scalp
    iii. nails – brittle
    iv.   xanthoma – rare
3. Cushing's syndrome – uncommon
    i.   skin – striae, thin skin, purpura – all related to abnormal collagen, pityriasis vesicolor
    ii.   hair – some hirsutes
    iii. acne – pustules and papules; common
    iv.   hyperpigmentation – an increase in MSH-like activity
    v.   subcutaneous fat – truncal obesity with thin limbs, buffalo hump
4. Acromegaly – rare
    i.   skin – coarse, thick, greasy
    ii.   hair – hirsutes
    iii. seborrhoea – frequent feature
5. Hypopituitarism – rare
    i.   skin – atrophied, thin, smooth, wrinkled, dry
    ii.   hair – loss of sexual hair
    iii. asebia – sebum production much reduced
    iv.   hypopigmentation – decrease in MSH peptides
6. Addison's disease – rare; hyperpigmentation – predilection for skin creases and light-exposed areas

Skin manifestations of ulcerative colitis

1. Aphthous ulcers – 10 per cent of patients
2. Erythema nodosum – 5–10 per cent of patients, may be recurrent
3. Perianal abscess and fistula – about 10 per cent of patients
4. Pyoderma gangrenosum <10 per cent of patients
5. Erythema multiforme – occasionally
6. Miscellaneous – cachexia, thrombophlebitis, signs of cirrhosis

Mucocutaneous features of SLE

Presented in decreasing order of frequency

1. Cutaneous vasculitis – often of fingers
2. Rash
   i. classical butterfly ⎫ in 60–70 per cent of all patients
   ii. livedo reticularis ⎭
3. Alopecia – diffuse or patchy; unrelated to disease activity
4. Aphthous ulcers   ⎫
5. Raynaud's phenomenon ⎬ 30 per cent of all patients
6. Photosensitivity to UV light ⎭
7. Purpura   ⎫
8. Subcutaneous nodules – elbows ⎬ in about 20 per cent of all patients
9. Discoid lesions   ⎭

Skin reactions to internal malignancy

1. Cachexia – pallor, fine thin dry skin, with reduced elasticity
2. Itch – particularly associated with lympho-reticular disease
3. Clubbing – lung cancer
4. Spontaneous venous thrombosis – occasional
5. Herpes zoster – relates to lympho-reticular malignancy
6. Dermatomyositis – up to 50 per cent of adults with this condition have cancer; rare. Carcinoma, leukaemia or lymphoma
7. Skin secondaries – most common in lung cancer
8. Acanthosis nigricans – gastric or bronchial carcinoma most common causes but a rare manifestation
9. Leukaemic infiltrate
10. Disseminated viral lesions secondary to immune paresis
11. Hypertrophic pulmonary osteo-arthropathy – lung cancer; rare
12. Flushing in carcinoid syndrome – rare

Causes of erythema nodosum

1. Sarcoid
2. Streptococcal infection
3. Inflammatory bowel disease
4. Tuberculosis
5. Sulphonamides, penicillin and salicylates
6. Behçet's disease
7. Isolated
8. Pregnancy and contraceptive pill

Chapter 19

Miscellaneous conditions

Paediatric diagnoses at a glance

The following conditions are sufficiently characteristic that a diagnosis may be confidently made after very brief inspection. They are not arranged in any order of frequency. These two lists are included to remind candidates of some diseases they may see as 'short cases'.

1. Down's syndrome – trisomy 21
2. Hypothyroidism
3. Turner's syndrome – XO
4. Nephrotic syndrome
5. Hurler's syndrome
6. Achondroplasia
7. Sturge–Weber syndrome
8. Adenoma sebaceum
9. Pierre Robin syndrome
10. Treacher-Collins syndrome
11. Craniosynostosis
12. Wardenberg's syndrome
13. Hydrocephalus
14. Hypercalcaemia
15. Albinism
16. Osteogenesis imperfecta

Adult diagnoses at a glance

1. Depression
2. Parkinson's disease
3. Blue bloater
4. Pink puffer
5. Myxoedema
6. Exophthalmos
7. Acne rosacea
8. Vitiligo
9. Polycythaemia

10. Malignant cachexia
11. SVC obstruction
12. Horner's syndrome
13. III or VII nerve palsy
14. Bell's palsy
15. Addisonian anaemia
16. Ophthalmic shingles
17. Progressive systemic sclerosis
18. Primary biliary cirrhosis
19. Xanthelasmata
20. Temporal arteritis
21. Rash of lupus
22. Alopecia areata
23. Myasthenia gravis
24. Dystrophia myotonica
25. Sjögren's syndrome
26. Dermatomyositis
27. Hereditary haemorrhagic telangiectasia
28. Peutz–Jeghers syndrome
29. Pseudoxanthoma elasticum
30. Cushing's syndrome
31. Acromegaly
32. Nelson's syndrome
33. Ochronosis
34. Haemochromatosis

Causes of nose bleeds

Usually from a vein just behind the columella in young people. In older patients the most usual site is the caudal nasal septum (Little's area), which is a region of multiple arterial anastomoses.

1. Trauma – sneezing, picking, injury
2. Degenerative arterial disease – also hypertension
3. Blood diseases
4. Local vascular malformations ⎫ infrequent
5. Superior mediastinal obstruction ⎭

Hypothermia

Core temperature <35°C (95°F)

DECREASED HEAT PRODUCTION

1. Hypothyroidism
2. Severe malnutrition

3. Inactivity
    i.   living alone
    ii. aged
    iii. crippled
    iv. depression
    v.   Parkinsonism

INCREASED HEAT LOSS

1. Exposure or lack of adequate garments
2. Prolonged alcoholic intoxication
3. Erythematous skin disease

FAILURE OF THERMOREGULATORY CONTROL

1. Any severe illness, especially in elderly
    i.   stroke
    ii. infection
    iii. heart failure
2. Drug overdose with coma

Complications of hypothermia

1. Cardiovascular
    i.   hypotension
    ii. bradyarrhythmias – J waves
    iii. ventricular fibrillation (often self-limiting)
2. Lung
    i.   bronchopneumonia
    ii. pulmonary oedema
    iii. hypoxia, hypercapnia
3. Metabolic
    i.   fluid shifts from vascular to interstitial spaces
    ii. metabolic acidosis
    iii. hypoglycaemia
4. Others
    i.   haemorrhagic pancreatitis
    ii. erosions of stomach or bowel
    iii. gastric or colonic dilation
    iv. DIC
    v.   miosis

Indications for CT scanning

GENERAL INDICATIONS

1. When a mass distorts the contour of an organ
2. To demonstrate a lesion with a different density from surrounding tissues
3. To differentiate between cysts and solid structures

Not of use in

1. Skeletal metastases – isotope scanning is better
2. Tumours within the gut – they are not well shown

INDICATIONS

1. CNS
   i.   primary and secondary neoplasms after CXR
   ii.   suspected SAH but aneurysms are not displayed unless large
   iii. head injury in unconscious patients with focal signs
   iv.   abscess, encephalitis, some cases of meningitis
   v.   to differentiate between stroke and tumour
   vi.   epilepsy of late origin
   vii. subdural haematoma
   viii. intra-orbital tumours
2. CVS
3. Respiratory system } *see* page 52
4. Abdomen
   i.   intra-abdominal masses – very accurate
   ii.   pancreatic masses
   iii. abdominal nodes – if enlarged
   iv.   liver metastases–but US very sensitive
5. Urogenital system
   i.   differentiation between kidney cysts and masses
   ii.   hydronephrosis – but well shown by IVU
   iii. renal calculi
   vi.   staging metastasized bladder cancer

Indications for bone scanning in patients with cancer

Radionuclide imaging is preferred before X-rays because a scan is more sensitive than radiology. In most cancers a negative scan virtually excludes the presence of metastases.

1. Staging of disease before therapy
2. Demonstrating occult metastases
3. Useful in areas which are radiologically 'difficult' – sternum, scapular and faciomaxillary regions
4. Confirm clinical suspicion of metastases
5. Monitoring effects of treatment
6. In lung cancer the presence of metastases precludes surgical cure

FALSE POSITIVES FOUND IN

1. Bone abscesses
2. Osteomalacia
3. Paget's disease of bone
4. Fractures

Pyrexia of unknown origin (PUO)

An unexplained fever, remittent or intermittent, which persists for more than 5–7 days

1. Infection
2. Malignancy
3. Drug hypersensitivity
4. Collagen vascular disease

while there are multiple causes of a PUO, these four groups of conditions cover about 80 per cent of cases

Adenocarcinoma from an unknown primary site

1. Lung
2. Colon
3. Pancreas
4. Liver

the most common origins; the prognosis is poor with a median survival of around three months

Causes of scoliosis (lateral curvature of spine)

NON-STRUCTURAL

1. Compensatory – secondary to a shortened leg
2. Sciatic – disc prolapse
3. Retroperitoneal abscess

STRUCTURAL

1. Idiopathic – 75 per cent of cases
2. Congenital – 15 per cent of cases

3. Neurological – 5 per cent of cases
    i.   secondary to UMN lesions – such as cerebral palsy
    ii. secondary to LMN lesions – polio or muscular dystrophy
4. Rheumatoid disease – not a severe scoliosis
5. Trauma
    i.   fracture
    ii. laminectomy
6. Infection of vertebra
7. Metabolic
    i.   rickets
    ii. homocystinuria
8. Neurofibromatosis
9. Marfan's syndrome

Causes of low back pain

1. Degenerative disorders
    i.   osteoarthritis
    ii. chronic disc herniation
    iii. spondylosis
2. Trauma
    i.   lumbar strain – very common
    ii. compression fracture of vertebral body
    iii. spondylolysis and spondylolisthesis
3. Tumours
    i.   metastases – breast, bronchus, prostate, kidney, thyroid
    ii. myeloma
    iii. neural tumours involving bone, nerve roots or meninges –
         uncommon
4. Inflammatory disease
    i.   rheumatoid arthritis – adult and juvenile
    ii. seronegative arthropathies – *see* page 274
5. Metabolic – osteoporosis
6. Infections
    i.   tuberculosis
    ii. chronic osteomyelitis
7. Abdominal aortic aneurysm
8. Compensation related

Frozen shoulder (adhesive capsulitis)

FEATURES

Increasing pain in and around the shoulder with loss of active and passive movements. Peak incidence – age 50–70 years. May last 1–2 years.

ASSOCIATED OR PRECIPITATING CAUSES

1. Hemiplegia – the most common
2. Trauma – particularly if kept immobile
3. Ischaemic heart disease
4. Thoracic surgery
5. Thyroid disease
6. Diabetes
7. Drugs – phenobarbitone, isoniazid

Common causes of painful knees

1. Osteoarthritis – the most common
2. Meniscal lesions – quite common
3. Ligamentous damage – common
4. Painful swollen joint – pus, blood or effusion
5. Rheumatoid arthritis
6. Patello-femoral osteoarthritis
7. Chondromalacia patellae – young adults ⎱ relatively
8. Osteochondritis dissecans – older children ⎰ common

Common causes of neck pain

1. Degenerative
    i.   cervical spondylosis
    ii. cervical disc lesions
2. Secondary (and occasional primary) tumours
3. Inflammatory
    i.   rheumatoid arthritis
    ii. seronegative arthritides especially ankylosing spondylitis
    iii. juvenile chronic rheumatoid
    iv. infection
4. Trauma
    i.   fracture
    ii. whiplash injury
5. Cervical rib
6. Non-specific
    i.   soft-tissue rheumatism
    ii. postural
    iii. fibrositis

Causes of pain around the elbow

1. Muscle pain – tennis elbow; tearing of extensor fibres at their insertion
2. Olecranon bursitis
3. Various fractures
4. Ulnar neuritis
5. Impaction of radial head – usually caused by swinging young children by their arms
6. Rheumatoid arthritis

Causes of restless legs syndrome

1. Rheumatoid arthritis (one-third of patients)
2. Pregnancy
3. Iron deficiency anaemia
4. Uraemia
5. Diabetes mellitus
6. Smoking
7. Parkinson's disease
8. Avitaminosis
9. Poliomyelitis

Comparison of attempted suicide and 'true' suicide

TABLE 19.1

	Attempted suicide	Suicide
Frequency	About 30 times more frequent than suicide. Increasing	Steady rate
Age	Younger > older	Older > younger
Sex	Females > males	Males > females
Marital status	Divorced and single	Widowed, divorced or single
Social isolation	Unrelated	Related
Employment	More frequent in unemployment	Retired and unemployed
Dwelling place	Poor inner city areas > rural areas	Commoner in cities
Technique	Benzodiazepines, analgesics antidepressants or mixtures	Barbiturates } often with alcohol
Alcohol	Often associated	Often associated
Pre-suicide personality	Much less often depressed Tend to be maladjusted	Often depressed, previously well adjusted
Outcome	Rarely fatal	May well be fatal

Effects of a high dose of radiation

EARLY

1. >5000 rads in 48 hours – delirium, ataxia, respiratory distress and death
2. Lower doses
   i.   nausea, vomiting, malaise with later relapse
   ii. diarrhoea
   iii. neutropenia and thrombocytopenia
   iv. alopecia
   v.   sterility

LATE

1. Cataracts
2. Leukaemia
3. Retarded development of unborn children
4. Infertility in men

Prognosis in severe shock

Outcome relates more closely to the duration of shock than to its severity. Septic shock has a mortality of at least 50 per cent.

ADVERSE FEATURES

1. Cardiac failure
2. Respiratory failure, especially ARDS – *see* page 46
3. Renal failure
4. Clouding of consciousness
5. Persistent jaundice
6. Increasing age
7. Sepsis
8. Oxygen consumption $<120\,ml$/minute per m^2 (normal $300\,ml$/minute per m^2)
9. Development of pulmonary hypertension
10. Laboratory findings
    i.   raised partial thromboplastin time
    ii. persistent thrombocytopenia
    iii. endotoxaemia
    iv. complement activation

Multiple organ failure

1. Sepsis – the most common cause
2. Major trauma
3. Extensive burns
4. Major surgery

Blood cultures are usually negative due to the use of prophylactic antibiotics. Thus a focus of sepsis may produce acute or chronic endotoxaemia in the absence of bacteraemia. The clinical features are very similar to the above list of adverse features in severe shock with the addition of

1. Acute right heart failure – secondary to pulmonary hypertension
2. Defective reticulo-endothelial function
3. Sub-nourishment
4. Immune deficiency
5. Relative deficiency of cortisol production and abnormalities of pituitary and thyroid function
6. Encephalopathy.

Alcohol and disease

Per capita spending and consumption continues to increase while the relative cost of alcohol falls. The pleasurable effects of drinking may encourage a person to drink more frequently and liberally with transition to regular drinking, habituation, dependence and compulsive drinking.

1. There is probably no true 'safe' level of drinking
2. Units of alcohol
   Half a pint of beer or lager = 1 glass of wine = 1 small sherry = 1 measure of vermouth or aperitif = 1 single gin or whisky. Consensus of views holds that 21 units for a man and 14 for a woman per week is safe, whereas >50 or 35 respectively is definitely harmful
3. Daily alcohol is more likely to be harmful than intermittent drinking
4. Generally women achieve higher blood alcohol concentrations than men for the same dose: women are smaller than men, ethanol is distributed in total body water and has zero order kinetics (see page 308).
5. Any drinking before driving impairs judgement. At the legal limit of blood alcohol (80 mg/100 ml) the chance of a driving accident is increased by a factor of 2–4. With higher plasma ethanol concentrations the probability of accident multiplies.
6. The only safe alcohol intake in pregnancy is zero.

CONSEQUENCES OF ALCOHOLISM

Medical

1. Chronic gastritis
2. Peptic ulcer
3. Alcoholic hepatitis, cirrhosis and hepatoma in 15 per cent of alcoholic cirrhotics
4. Varices and bleeding
5. Reactive hypoglycaemia
6. Recurrent pancreatitis
7. Macrocytosis
8. Vitamin deficiency
9. Pneumonia
10. Tuberculosis
11. Impotence
12. Peripheral neuropathy
13. Alcohol amblyopia
14. Wernicke–Korsakoff syndrome

all effects of sub-nutrition (1 g ethanol contains 30 kJ energy and no protein)

15. Suicide
16. Hyperlipidaemia (Type IV)
17. Hyperuricaemia
18. Alcoholic ketoacidosis
19. Fetal alcohol syndrome
20. Morning anorexia, nausea and vomiting
21. Hypertension
22. Cardiomyopathy

Acute events

1. Acute alcohol poisoning
2. Acute gastritis
3. Acute trauma
4. Peripheral nerve pressure palsies
5. Amnesia

Psychological consequences

1. Anxiety and depression
2. Trauma
3. Hallucinations
4. Paranoid states
5. Delirium tremens
6. Other drug abuse
7. Sexual difficulties
8. Impaired memory and concentration

Social consequences
1. Aggression and domestic violence
2. Child neglect or abuse
3. Debt
4. Family difficulties
5. Social isolation
6. Absenteeism
7. Homelessness
8. Stigma of dependence

Legal features
1. Driving offences
2. Drunk and disorderly
3. Criminal damage
4. Theft
5. Vagrancy

Cannabis

The psychotropic effects result from limbic localization of Δ^9-tetrahydrocannabinol. The limbic system is the motivational centre of the brain and is involved with memory, cognition and psychomotor performance. The drugs crosses the placenta and enters breast milk.

EFFECTS OF CANNABINOIDS

1. Psychotropic
2. Hypnotic
3. Tranquillizing
4. Anti-emetic
5. Analgesic
6. Lowers intraocular pressure
7. Increases appetite
8. Cardiovascular – tachycardia, hypotension, hypertension
9. Inhibits T-cell function

Risks of oral contraception

Mortality – rare; but there is an excess annual mortality rate from the following

1. Peripheral venous thrombosis
2. Thromboembolism
3. Myocardial infarction
4. Cerebrovascular lesions

Morbidity – infrequent, considering the large numbers of women taking the pill

1. CVS
    i.   as for 1–4 in Mortality
    ii. hypertension – slow rise, potentially reversible
2. Metabolic
    i.   impaired glucose tolerance
    ii. increase in cholesterol and triglycerides
    iii. increase in gall bladder disease
    iv. drug interactions – antibiotics, rifampicin, phenytoin
3. Neoplasia – hepatoma; rare
4. Urinary tract infections – more common in pill users

Return of fertility
1. Cervical erosions – easily treated
2. Post-pill anovulation – delayed return
3. Irregular menstruation

Oestrogen therapy

BENEFITS

1. Hot flushes
2. Vaginal atrophy   } reduction in
3. Rate of bone loss

DISADVANTAGES

1. Tender breasts
2. Nausea and vomiting
3. Breakthrough bleeding

HAZARDS

1. Endometrial cancer
2. Gall-bladder disease
3. Possible thrombo-embolic disease

CONTRA-INDICATIONS

1. Oestrogen dependent neoplasia, past or
   present
2. Vaginal bleeding – undiagnosed   } absolute
3. History of thrombo-embolic disease

4. Heavy smoking
5. Uterine fibroids
6. Obesity   } relative
7. Hypertension
8. Diabetes
9. Severe varicose veins

Incubation and isolation of various common infections

TABLE 19.2

Disease	Incubation (days)		Isolation
	Usual	*Range*	
Chickenpox	14–15	(7–21)	1 week after appearance of rash
Rubella	14–18	(14–20)	Until rash fades
Mumps	17–18	(12–21)	Not less than 2 weeks from onset
Measles	10–11	(7–14)	For 5 days from beginning of rash
Pertussis	7–10		2 weeks after cough with whoop has ceased
Enteric fevers	2–21		Until 3 negative stool cultures
Poliomyelitis	7–14	(5–21)	3–4 weeks
Hepatitis A	4–6 weeks	2–6 weeks	7–12 days
Hepatitis B	3 months	6 weeks–6 months	Until patient becomes HB$_s$Ag negative
Hepatitis non-A non-B	6 weeks–3 months		Not known

Hepatitis B

High rates of infection in
1. Homosexual men
2. Prostitutes
3. Drug addicts

Groups at risk of infection
1. Patients requiring multiple transfusions (but all blood now screened in GB for HBV)
2. Patients with immune deficiencies
3. Patients with malignant disease
4. Staff on oncology units
5. Staff of mental institutions
6. Laboratory personnel

Vaccination recommended in
1. Staff of hepatitis reference laboratories
2. Staff of liver and oncology units
3. Dental nurses and surgeons
4. Immediate contacts of patients with thalassaemia or haemophilia – multiple transfusions
5. Sexual contacts of patients with acute hepatitis B

The major tropical diseases

1. Malaria
2. Schistosomiasis
3. Filariasis – including onchocerciasis
4. Trypanosomiasis – African sleeping sickness and Chagas' disease
5. Leishmaniasis – visceral and mucocutaneous
6. Giardiasis
7. Amoebiasis
8. Leprosy

} may well be increasing because of undernutrition, overpopulation, poverty, poor hygiene, inadequate medical services, political instability; all militate against control

9. Poliomyelitis
10. Cholera
11. Yellow fever
12. Tuberculosis

} contained or treatable

Hazards of untreated milk

1. Bovine tuberculosis
2. Brucellosis

} eradicated from British herds

3. Salmonella
4. Enteropathic *Escherichia coli*
5. *Campylobacter* spp
6. Paratyphoid
7. Q fever

Some fevers in people coming from abroad
TABLE 19.3

Fever	Countries where infection may occur
1. Malaria – the most common	Many tropical countries
2. Typhoid – *Salmonella typhi*	Countries with poor sanitation
3. Hepatitis A and B	Related to poor sanitation and hygiene
4. Trypanosomiasis } Safari	East and Central Africa
5. Tick typhus } holidays	South and East Africa
6. Dengue and sandfly fevers	Mediterranean littoral, Middle-East, India, Caribbean and S. America
7. Kala-azar	East Asia, S. America, Southern-half of Africa
8. Poliomyelitis	All tropical countries
9. Tuberculosis	Primarily in people arriving from developing countries
10. Yellow fever	Central and W. Africa, Central and S. America

ESSENTIAL QUESTIONS

1. Areas visited, activities undertaken
2. Which immunizations received before travelling?
3. Any untreated water drunk?
4. History of contacts
5. Illnesses of other members of the party
6. Any casual sexual contacts?

Infections that may be caught from animals (zoonoses)

TABLE 19.4

Disease	Infective agent	Animal
Psittacosis	*Chlamydia*	Budgerigars, parrots, pigeons
Brucellosis	*Brucella melitensis*	Sheep, goats
	B. abortus	Cattle
	B. suis	Pigs
Leptospirosis	*Leptospira*	Small domestic and wild animals
Orf	Poxvirus	Sheep and goats
Anthrax	*Bacillus anthracis* (spores)	Sheep, cattle and dried skins thereof

CANINE ZOONOSES

1. Wound sepsis involving *Pasteurella multocida*
2. Toxocara infestations
3. *Campylobacter jejuni* enteritis
4. Ringworm
5. Arthropod infestation

Noises in the neck

1. Cervical venous hum – continuous, heard above medial ends of clavicles and anterior border of sternomastoid muscle
    i.   usually of no importance
    ii. high output states
2. Bruits transmitted via carotid arteries
    i.   aortic stenosis
    ii. mitral regurgitation
3. Bruits from carotid arteries – usually implies that the patient has generalized vascular disease
    i.   atherosclerosis – frequent disease
4. Murmurs from overactive thyroid glands – rare

Side effects of corticosteroids

Occur primarily from oral use but also from prolonged topical application. The effects are proportional to the dose and length of treatment.

METABOLIC CONSEQUENCES

1. Mineralocorticoid effects
   i.   sodium and water retention, potassium loss
   ii. hypertension
   iii. thinning of skin, striae
   iv. moon face
   v.   central obesity

2. Glucocorticoid effects
   i.   diabetes mellitus
   ii. hyperlipidaemia

3. Catabolic effects
   i.   myopathy
   ii. osteoporosis
   iii. aseptic bone necrosis

4. Modification of natural responses
   i.   suppression of fever, inflammation, pain and ESR
   ii. increased chance of infection
   iii. delayed wound healing

5. Miscellaneous
   i.   acne, hypertrichosis
   ii. dyspepsia, peptic ulceration
   iii. euphoria
   iv. psychosis
   v.   growth retardation in children
   vi. cataracts
   vii. the children of pregnant women taking steroid hormones may have a cleft palate or congenital cataract

SUPPRESSION OF THE HYPOTHALAMIC—PITUITARY—ADRENAL AXIS

1. Adrenal atrophy
2. Danger of Addisonian crisis
3. Pigmentation

Contra-indications to the use of anticoagulants

1. Active gut ulcer
2. Infective endocarditis
3. Non-embolic cerebrovascular accidents
4. Severe hepatic insufficiency
5. Recent injury or surgery to eye or CNS
6. Alcoholism
7. Haemostatic defect – ? excluding DIC
8. More than 70 or so years of age

Complications of enteral nutrition

1. Local
    i.   oesophagitis
    ii. oesophageal erosions or stricture
2. Gastrointestinal
    i.   diarrhoea – very common
    ii. abdominal distension and pain
3. Metabolic
    i.   hyperglycaemia
    ii. hypokalaemia
    iii. hypocalcaemia
    iv. hypophosphataemia
    v.   reduced serum Zn^{2+} and Mg^{2+}
4. Non-specific liver function abnormalities
5. Pneumonitis from aspiration of feeds

The metabolic complications of parenteral nutrition are similar to those of enteral nutrition.

Common X-linked disorders

Listed in descending order down the X genome

1. Duchenne muscular dystrophy
2. Becker muscular dystrophy
3. Chronic granulomatous disease
4. Retinitis pigmentosa
5. Alport's syndrome
6. Agammaglobulinaemia
7. Fabry's disease
8. Hunter syndrome

 9. Haemophilia B
10. G6PD deficiency
11. Favism
12. Haemophilia A

Pharmacokinetics

Factors concerned in drug disposition

1. Absorption
2. Lipid/water solubility
3. Serum protein binding
4. Tissue binding
5. Pathways of metabolism
6. Biliary, renal (and lung) excretion
7. Age

> all may well
> be altered in
> ill people

Factors causing decline in drug concentration in plasma

1. Uptake by liver and elimination in bile
2. Removal of glomerular filtration
3. Removal by tubular secretion
4. Metabolism
5. Uptake into tissues – normally
    a reversible process

> not reversible; rate
> of removal
> proportional to
> drug concentration

Efficacy and potency

Efficacy is the ability of a drug to produce its maximum therapeutic effect – a measure of the maximum obtainable effect. Thus heroin is a more effective analgesic than aspirin.

Potency is a measure of the amount of drug required to produce a given effect. Bumetanide (1 mg) is more potent than frusemide (40 mg) but this does not mean that bumetanide is more effective than frusemide. Potency is therefore not relevant to the clinical effectiveness of a drug.

Potentiation and synergism

Potentiation occurs when the effect of two or more drugs in combination is greater than the sum of their individual effects. Alcohol enhances the effects of diazepam, and rifampicin inhibits hepatic metabolism of warfarin increasing the anticoagulant effect.

These are examples of pharmacodynamic potentiation and pharmacokinetic interaction, respectively.

Synergism is chiefly used in the context of antibiotics. Thus the combination of flucloxacillin and gentamicin is synergistic against streptococci.

Volume of distribution (V_D)

Total amount of drug in body at zero time × volume in which drug is distributed. V_D does not necessarily reflect a literal volume of fluid in which the drug is dissolved.

Plasma half-life ($T_{1/2}$)

The time taken for the concentration of a drug in blood or plasma to decline to half of its original value.

Drug clearance

The volume of blood or plasma cleared of a drug in a unit time. Related to V_D, $T_{1/2}$ or to the elimination constant K_{el}.

Thus: $C\ell_p = V_D \times K_{el}$

Clearance is the sum of individual clearance values – e.g. renal, hepatic and metabolic (degradation) clearances

Area under the curve (AUC)

The intensity and duration of a tissue response to a drug is often a function of the concentration and persistence of the drug in blood or plasma. This response is related to AUC and AUC is closely related to drug clearance (ml/min). The bigger the AUC the smaller plasma clearance and hence a more prolonged action.

First pass effects

Drugs which are absorbed from the gut pass first through the liver. Metabolism of the drug may occur in the liver. This extraction of the drug before it reaches the systemic circulation is called the first pass effect.

First- and zero-order processes

When the rate of elimination of a drug depends upon its remaining concentration this is a first-order process. This removal increases in direct proportion to the plasma concentration. If a drug is removed independent of its concentration this is a zero-order process and is consequent upon saturation of the elimination process.

Alcohol is a good example of zero-order elimination; the plasma concentration falls by about 15–20 mg/100 ml per hour until the alcohol has been completely removed.

First-order processes may become zero-order when high drug concentrations are present. If therapy continues, drug accumulation and possible toxicity ensue.

Bioavailability and bioequivalence

Bioavailability is the amount of drug present in the body. Bioequivalence is concerned with the efficacy and includes factors such as rate of absorption, first-pass metabolism, peak plasma concentrations, penetration into tissues, duration of action and rate of removal. Two drugs may have similar bioavailability, but differ importantly in efficacy.

Receptors, agonists and antagonists

RECEPTOR

An area of a cellular membrane or intracellular protein capable of binding endogenous substances or members of a specific group of drugs. The binding leads to some change in function of the cell.

LIGAND

Any substance which binds to a receptor.

AGONIST

A ligand which produces an appropriate response when bound to its receptor.

ANTAGONIST

A ligand which prevents the effects of an agonist. Pure antagonists produce no effect when receptor bound.

PARTIAL AGONIST (OR PARTIAL ANTAGONIST)

A ligand which is a pure agonist (or antagonist) at low concentrations but which at higher concentrations has some agonist (or antagonist) properties.

'UP-REGULATION' AND 'DOWN-REGULATION'

These terms indicate increase (or decrease) in the number of receptor sites. Such changes occur in response to long-term administration of a drug (the dose of which may then need to be increased) and in diseases.

Adverse drug reactions

Type A – those to be expected from the pharmacological properties of the drug such as bleeding from an excess of warfarin. Morbidity high, mortality low

Type B – unexpected, less common than Type A but have a greater morbidity and mortality

PATIENTS AT HIGHER THAN AVERAGE CHANCE OF AN ADVERSE REACTION
1. Women > men
2. Elderly
3. People receiving multiple drugs
4. Patients with cancer
5. Patients with renal impairment
6. Patients receiving drugs from two different doctors

THE MOST COMMON DRUGS IMPLICATED

1. Aspirin
2. Digoxin
3. Diuretics
4. Antibiotics
5. Anticoagulants
6. Corticosteroids
7. Cytotoxic drugs

Some epidemiological definitions

RATES

The numbers of people with a disease or numbers of events births, hospital admissions, deaths, etc.) in relation to the total population at risk. Rates have a time limit, a *numerator* (the number of cases of a disease or events) and a *denominator* (the population). Populations are specifically defined groups of people in terms of age, sex or occupation. *Crude rates* are not standardized for age, sex or other variables.

MORTALITY STATISTICS

Derived from death certificates and allow general trends in disease pattern to be identified.

OCCUPATIONAL MORTALITY

The recording of the occupation of the deceased on death registration allows the identification of high risk occupations such as deep sea diving or coal mining.

MORBIDITY STATISTICS

Relatively imprecise information is obtained from

1. Hospital inpatient statistics at the time of discharge but no records of outpatient diagnoses are easily available
2. Inpatient statistics from the Mental Health Enquiry. Periodic reports are issued
3. Notifications of quarantinable, infectious and parasitic diseases. Changes in the number of notifications may reflect changes in frequency
4. Cancer registration
5. Social Security statistics – give a general guide as to the frequency of causes of absence from work

PREVALENCE

The proportion of people in a population who are affected by a disease at one particular time.

INCIDENCE

The number of new cases of a disease in a population in a given period of time.

CROSS-SECTIONAL AND LONGITUDINAL STUDIES

For a cross-sectional study, a defined population is investigated at one point in time which gives the prevalence. When a cohort of people is studied more than once, the incidence and possible aetiological factors are noted. This is a longitudinal study.

STANDARDIZED MORTALITY RATIO

An age and sex standardized rate which is used because of the uneven distribution of disease between sexes and at different ages and between one population and another.

ANALYTICAL STUDIES

1. Case-control studies compare people with a disease and those without it
2. Cohort studies compare people exposed to the suspected cause and those not exposed

Index